# Optimizing the Process of Teaching English for Medical Purposes with the Use of Mobile Applications

# POLISH STUDIES IN ENGLISH LANGUAGE AND LITERATURE

Edited by Jacek Fisiak



VOL. 39

PETER LANG
EDITION

Maria Chojnacka

# Optimizing the Process of Teaching English for Medical Purposes with the Use of Mobile Applications

## A Memrise-based Case Study

PETER LANG
EDITION

**Bibliographic Information published by the Deutsche Nationalbibliothek**
The Deutsche Nationalbibliothek lists this publication in the Deutsche Nationalbibliografie; detailed bibliographic data is available in the internet at http://dnb.d-nb.de.

This publication was financially supported by the University of Social Sciences in Warsaw.

Library of Congress Cataloging-in-Publication Data
A CIP catalog record for this book has been applied for at the Library of Congress

ISSN 1436-7513
ISBN 978-3-631-73061-4 (Print)
E-ISBN 978-3-631-73062-1 (E-PDF)
E-ISBN 978-3-631-73063-8 (EPUB)
E-ISBN 978-3-631-73064-5 (MOBI)
DOI 10.3726/b11583

Peter Lang Edition is an Imprint of Peter Lang GmbH.

Peter Lang – Frankfurt am Main · Bern · Bruxelles · New York · Oxford · Warszawa · Wien


This publication has been peer reviewed.

www.peterlang.com

# Table of Contents

# List of tables

# List of figures

# List of abbreviations

| | |
|---|---|
| AIDS | Acquired Immune Deficiency Syndrome |
| ALTE | Association for Language Testers in Europe |
| APGAR | Appearance, Pulse, Grimace, Activity, Regulation |
| AWL | Academic Word List |
| BE | Basic English |
| BULATS | Business Language Testing Service |
| BYOD | Bring Your Own Device |
| BYOP | Bring Your Own Phone |
| CABG | Coronary Artery Bypass Grafting |
| CALL | Computer Assisted Language Learning |
| CDA | Critical Discourse Analysis |
| CEFR | Common European Framework of Reference |
| CHOP | Cyclophosphamide Hydroxydaunomycin, Oncovin, and Prednisone |
| DNA | Deoxyribonucleic Acid |
| EABP | English for Academic Business Purposes |
| EALP | English for Academic Legal Purposes |
| EAMP | English for Academic Medical Purposes |
| EAP | English for Academic Purposes |
| EBP | English for Business Purposes |
| EGAP | English for General Academic Purposes |
| EGBP | English for General Business Purposes |
| EGP | English for General Purposes |
| ELP | English for Legal Purposes |
| ELT | English Language Teaching |
| EMP | English for Medical Purposes |
| EOP | English for Occupational Purposes |
| ESAP | English for Specific Academic Purposes |
| ESBP | English for Specific Business Purposes |
| ESCP | English for Sociocultural Purposes |
| ESP | English for Specific Purposes |
| EST | English for Science and Technology |
| EVP | English for Vocational Purposes |
| FME | Fundamental Medical English |
| GE | General English |

| | |
|---|---|
| GMC | General Medical Council |
| GMER | Global Minimum Essential Requirements |
| GP | General Practitioner |
| IELTS | International English Language Testing System |
| IATEFL | International Association of English as a Foreign Language |
| IBS | Irritable Bowel Syndrome |
| ICD | International Classification of Diseases |
| ICFE | International Certificate in Financial English |
| ILEC | International Legal English Certificate |
| IMG | International Medical Graduate |
| IMR(A)D | Introduction, Methods, Results, and Discussion |
| JEAP | Journal of English for Academic Purposes |
| JSLW | Journal of Second Language Writing |
| KWIC | Key Word in Context |
| LTM | Long Term Memory |
| LSP | Language for Specific Purposes |
| MALL | Mobile Assisted Language Learning |
| MALU | Mobile Assisted Language Use |
| MAWL | Medical Academic Word List |
| MBL | Mobile Based Learning |
| MMEC | Mobile Medical English Companion |
| MRA | Medical Research Articles |
| OET | Occupational English Test |
| PLAB | Professional and Linguisitc Assessment Board |
| PROFEX | Proficiency Examination of English for Medical Purposes |
| RBC | Red Blood Cell |
| RDC | Responsive Course Design |
| ROHHAD | Rapid-Onset Obesity with Hypothalamic Dysfunction, Hypoventilation and Autonomic Dysregulation |
| SARS | Severe Acute Respiratory Syndrome |
| SME | Specialized Medical English |
| SRS | Spaced Repetition Software |
| sTANDEM | Standardised Language Certificate for Medical Purposes |
| USMLE | United States Medical Licensing Examination |
| TESOL | Teachers of English to Speakers of Other Languages Association |
| WBC | White Blood Cell |

# Introduction

Challenges to Language for Specific Purposes (LSP) pedagogy have received a lot of attention among researchers, with the first research accounts dating from 1960s. Presently, a comprehensive account of approaches towards LSP methodology can be found in a wide array of publications, e.g. Paltridge – Starfield (2013) or Gajewska – Sowa (2014), among the most recent ones. English for Specific Purposes is by far the fastest growing and the most common branch of LSP, e.g. there are over one hundred ESP coursebooks aimed at specific disciplines available from one of the biggest international publishing houses. An increasing number of universities offer courses, or even entire study programs in ESP. There also exist well-established, peer-reviewed ESP-dedicated journals and vigorous ESP communities are mushrooming throughout the world.

The ubiquity of mobile devices has opened the way to extending learning environments far beyond the constraints of the traditional foreign language classroom. The concepts of m-learning, mobile assisted language learning (MALL) or mobile assisted language use (MALU) have also received pronounced research attention, which has led to an ever-increasing number of publications regarding the use of mobile technologies in foreign language teaching (e.g. Gajek 2015, among the most recent publications). World-wide telecollaboration projects, or publications in peer-reviewed journals dedicated to e-, m- or u- learning are the bread and butter of the vigorous digital communities.

Studies have been undertaken to investigate the domains of English for Specific Purposes or the domain of mobile learning, yet there are only a few studies regarding the learning and teaching of English for Medical Purposes (EMP) as a domain of ESP, but supported by mobile environments. And it is the merger of good EMP practice with the ubiquitous and dynamic nature of mobile learning that lies at the heart of this book as a proper understanding of the mechanisms leading to the efficacy or lack of it in the case of mobile supported EMP language use is an important determinant and predictor of learner success or failure.

This book seeks to advance the knowledge about effective learning and teaching of English for Medical Purposes to medical students. The analysis of empirical data is preceded by theoretical considerations of the current state of research in the field. The author seeks to investigate the effectiveness of the use of a mobile version of a flashcard spaced-repetition learning platform (Memrise.com) to support the learning of English for Medical Purposes. Yet the ultimate goal is to present a novel educational solution that supports the ongoing and situated learning of English for Medical Purposes.

**Chapter 1** provides an overview of concepts pertaining to the field of English for Specific Purposes. It characterises approaches towards the classification of languages for specific purposes and resultant pedagogical approaches. Moreover, it addresses the theoretical frameworks and developments in domain-related research over the centuries, with special focus on the convergence of ESP theory, research, and pedagogical practice. **Chapter 2** gives an insight into the domain of English for Medical Purposes as a sub-domain of English for Specific Purposes. It outlines core features of English for Medical Purposes and continues with a discussion of specialist language proficiency. **Chapter 3** focuses on the notions of motivation and learner autonomy in foreign language learning, with special focus on motivational theories relating to mobile learning environments. The unique role of the teacher in English for Medical Purposes training is acknowledged, however, the importance of self-directed learning and attitudes towards the use of technology are emphasised as important indicators of success or failure in mastering course content. This chapter lays out the theoretical foundations propelling the research project. As regards **Chapter 4**, it briefly sketches the current state of mobile learning theories, research and practice to focus on the nature of mobile assisted language learning and its unique benefits. The functionality of various types of intelligent flashcard vocabulary trainers and spaced-repetition software are discussed in the context of shaping the tools for learning English for Medical Purposes. The chapter continues with a detailed analysis of the features of Memrise – an online flashcard learning tool – which was used in the research project. It concludes with a review of projects involving the use of technology in teaching English for Medical Purposes. **Chapter 5** commences with the presentation of the research goals and the research method. The data collection instruments and procedures are outlined and a statistical analysis of the obtained data is presented. On the one hand, the research project aimed at determining to what extent medical students are open to the use of mobile technology in learning English for Medical Purposes. On the other hand, the author aimed to assess the effectiveness of Memrise as a learning tool in the context of specialist language. The findings are presented in relation to the research questions. Also, the limitations of the study are acknowledged. Finally, propelled by insights from the research project, **Chapter 6** is devoted to the presentation of a novel educational solution supporting the learning of English for Medical Purposes by medical students, i.e. a mobile spaced-repetition medical vocabulary tutor – the Mobile Medical English Companion (MMEC). The chapter explores the issues of its design and core principles.

# Chapter One: An Overview of Key Concepts Pertaining to Teaching English for Specific Purposes

## 1.1 Introduction

Broadly speaking, English for Specific Purposes (ESP) is an *umbrella* term used in association with both teaching and learning domain-driven English (Paltridge – Starfield 2013: 2, Orr 2002). The concept is far from new, as English can be traced back through history as the language of trade and science, yet most research in ESP dates back to the post-war period, especially the 1960s, when it became apparent that general English courses often failed to meet the needs and wants of specific groups of learners, especially in the workplace context (Hutchinson – Waters 1987: 5; Dudley-Evans – St John 1998: I, Brunton 2009: 1).

In the 21st century, one might assume that hoping for a clear-cut definition of the concept of ESP is not completely unwarranted. However, finding a viable definition of ESP still forms the background to much academic discussion. There is much disagreement over the scope of ESP, what it is, is not or should be. On one side of the spectrum, there is the position that language is always used for a specific purpose, and when it comes to teaching and learning English, "[e]very language course should be considered a course for specific purposes" (Douglas 2013: 368, after Long 2005: 1). On the other side of the spectrum, there are researchers who deny the existence of even the very concept of ESP.

The literature on ESP offers a broad selection of its types. The most commonly encountered acronyms (Belcher 2009a: 2–3) comprise English for Academic Purposes (EAP) and English for Occupational Purposes (EOP), with numerous subcategories available along a wide spectrum of specificity. Starting from the more general, one can find courses in English for Business Purposes (EBP), English for Legal Purposes (ELP) or English for Medical Purposes (EMP), or more specific, English for Stockbrokers, English for Forensics, English for Dentistry, English for Aviation and Air-traffic Controllers, English for the Military, English for Tourist Guides, English for Horse Breeders or English for Brewers, to mention just a few. This wide spectrum of specificity is clearly visible in textbook content, e.g. Oxford University Press offers well over one hundred ESP coursebooks ranging in specificity.

What seems to unite different these different types of ESP is "commitment to the purposes of the learners themselves" (Belcher 2009a: 3). Recently, maybe due to the "publish or perish" tendency, requiring non-native authors to publish papers and deliver presentations in English, the domain of ESP has witnessed an increase in interest in the merger of English for Academic Purposes (EAP) with English for Occupational Purposes (EOP) courses, leading to courses in English for Academic Business Purposes (EABP), English for Academic Legal Purposes (EALP) or English for Academic Medical Purposes (EAMP). English for Sociocultural Purposes (ESCP) seems to be yet another vigorously developing branch of ESP.

Despite differences in the theoretical accounts offered, what researchers do seem to be unanimous about is the fact that ESP learners are, most often, adults "facing a particular workplace, academic, or professional context" (Basturkmen – Elder 2004: 672–673) and that despite varying contexts (Basturkmen 2006: ix), there always exists a specific target-group of learners with specific communicative needs (Paltridge – Starfield 2013: 2).

## 1.2 To ESP or not to ESP

It is critical to point out that a wide array of researchers refute the existence of the concept of ESP, whereas others refute the existence of the concept of *General English* (Johns – Price-Machado 2001: 44) or *English for No Obvious Reason* (Johns et al. 2011). Basturkmen argues that:

> "It can be argued that language varieties are based in and extend from a common core of language. Or it can be argued that language varieties are self-contained entities."
>
> (Basturkmen 2006: 28)

Bloor and Bloor (1986; in Basturkmen 2006: 15) discuss two approaches: the *Common Core Plus* and *No Common Core* approach to language. The former assumes the existence of a basic core of general language and its extension in the form of a particular specific-purpose language. The latter denies the existence of a single general-purpose variety of language. Following Bloor and Bloor (1986, in Basturkmen 2006: 17), there is no such thing as *General English*, since all language serves some specific purpose and is learned in a specific context. No language is used in a contextual void and every situation is a specific situation. Hence, it is possible to learn the common elements simultaneously with situation-specific items and even beginner learners might benefit from ESP instruction. There is no need to wait until they have mastered the "core". Bloor and Bloor, however, acknowledge the fact that some of those "varieties" may "overlap".

Grucza (2013a: 21–22) provides yet another classification of languages for specific purposes within which "language for specific purposes" is a subcategory of "language for general purposes", just like "dialects" or "sociolects". However,

Grucza (2013a, 2013b) highlights the fact that neither assuming the "coordinate" relationship between GE and LSP, nor assuming the "subordinate" relationship between GE and LSP is right, and the hierarchical approach should be abandoned as GE and LSP are not compatible but complementary, and to a great extent should be treated as distinct, and a native speaker of Polish knowing both "Polish for General Purposes" and some variety of "Polish for Specific Purposes" should be treated as bilingual.

Dudley-Evans and St John (1998: 8) suggest that there exists a "continuum" with General English (GE) and highly specific ESP located on the both sides of the spectrum. Also, following Quirk et al. (1972, in Basturkmen 2006: 15–16), Basturkmen argues for the existence of a common-core-general-purpose language used across life situations, consisting of high frequency items, and that learners first need to master the core and only later situation-specific items. Basturkmen (2006: 9) compares GE and ESP teaching to a voyage, the former resembling more Columbus's discoveries, the latter being made by ferry, where you know the exact destination point before you embark.

From a more practical angle, some of the dilemmas inherent in this framework concern the issue of "ultimate proficiency". Despite the Common European Framework of Reference (CEFR), it is indeed difficult to determine where the C2 level of General English starts and where it ends. How native-like should learners be for General English training to end? How many collocations should they know? Would these collocations embrace workplace jargon?

ESP on the other hand, focuses on reaching more clearly defined objectives in the most efficient way, with the scope of language to be mastered being to a greater extent secondary to specific domain-driven needs. Yet, although such a powerful educational device as easily defined objectives seems to be more at hand in ESP, Basturkmen does acknowledge the fact that even in ESP teaching there seems to be much disagreement over the "location" of this final endpoint.

In a similar vein, Ferris (2001, in Basturkmen – Elder 2004: 676) discusses the efficiency of two approaches to teaching English for Academic Purposes. One is the top-down approach – to teach "generalized academic writing skills" hoping that learners would transfer the skills to particular academic disciplines. The other is a bottom-up solution – to start with "discipline specific instruction" as different groups of learners require different instruction.

Also, Hyland (2002, in Basturkmen – Elder 2004: 676) is of the opinion that "(…) generic labels such as scientific language, business English or academic skills, are misleading in that they disguise and misrepresent the discursive complexity and variation between how different groups in those broad bands use language and their aims in doing so." Samraj's study from 2002 (in Basturkmen –

Elder 2004: 676) seems to support Hyland's point of view. Samaraj performed an analysis of wildlife behaviour and conservation biology article introductions to discover that the two had a different schematic structure and the transfer of writing skills via the top-down approach would not be facilitated at all.

## 1.3 Characteristics of ESP

This section is intended to provide a review of the literature regarding the characteristics of ESP and their relevance to foreign language teaching. As mentioned above, there exist many parallel classifications of types of ESP. To mention just a few: Hutchinson and Waters (1987) provide a tree-diagram of various forms of ESP; Dudley-Evans and St John (1998) offer a categorization of the ESP movement; Johns and Price-Machado (2001: 43) talk of "a remarkable array of ESP courses offered throughout the world" and Belcher (2009a: 2) offers a broad selection of "seemingly endless acronyms generated by the various branches of ESP". The most commonly known types of ESP (Belcher 2009a: 2–3; Johns – Price-Machado 2001: 43; Basturkmen – Elder 2004: 673, Dudley-Evans – St John 1998: 5; Brunton 2009) comprise English for Academic Purposes (EAP) and English for Occupational Purposes (EOP), with numerous subcategories available along a wide spectrum of specificity.

ESP programmes often adapt to market needs, using the "job shadowing" phenomenon (Johns – Price-Machado 2001: 48), with modules created in response to a new type of job being available for a given community. One of the more prominent examples of this phenomenon was the mushrooming of courses of English or German for Nursing, when Poland entered the European Union and many nurses left to work in nursery homes in Germany, Sweden or the United Kingdom. Johns and Price-Machado (2001: 43; after Huang 1999) provide the example of the sudden increase in the number of ESP courses in relation to the general number of EFL courses in China due to the development of foreign trade, as well as the example of ESP courses in computer language for American prisoners (Johns – Price-Machado 2001: 44).

At this point it is important to remember that the issue of domain specificity has always been one of the most fundamental questions in the field of ESP teaching (Basturkmen – Elder 2004: 673–676). Whereas current ESP practitioners seem to be in agreement over the goal of ESP being "specific-learner-centred language instruction" (Belcher 2009a: 1–2), it is not quite as clear how to achieve that aim. Nor has it always been a "learner-centred" approach.

Hutchinson and Waters (1987: 6–8; Brunton 2009) identify three factors responsible for the development of ESP as a branch of ELT in the second half of the

20th century. Firstly, there was the dominance of English-speaking countries in post World War II scientific development, paired with the globalization of commerce (Dudley-Evans – St John 1998: 19; Flowerdew 2013: 340). Knowing a foreign language was no longer "a sign of well-rounded education" but an indispensable work-related skill. Secondly came the growing popularity of the communicative approach in ELT, and a growing awareness of the contextualisation of language and genre-specific discourse, which resulted in a number of research projects aimed at defining particular sub-genres of ESP. Thirdly, there was a shift in the teacher-centeredness paradigm due to developments in educational psychology, resulting in a more "learner-centred" approach to teaching. The intertwinement of post-war globalization, the expectations and demands of learners wishing to learn relevant language for a particular purpose and the developments in educational psychology served as lynchpins in the formation of ESP methodology as we know it today.

Six characteristics of ESP were put forward by Strevens (Johns – Price-Machado 2001: 44–45; after Strevens 1988). He enumerates four absolute characteristics of ESP, according to which it should: 1) be designed to meet the specific needs of the learner, 2) have content related to particular disciplines, occupations, or activities (i.e. in its themes and topics), 3) be centred on the language appropriate to these activities in terms of syntax, lexis, discourse, semantics and 4) be in contrast with General English. He also adds two variable characteristics of ESP according to which it is to be restricted as regards the language skills to be learnt (e.g. reading only), and not taught according to any preordained methodology.

Dudley-Evans and St John (1998: 4–5; also working from Strevens 1988) postulated a slightly different distinction listing only three absolute ESP characteristics: 1) ESP is defined to meet specific needs of the learner, 2) it makes use of the underlying methodology and activities of the discipline it serves and 3) it is centred on the language (grammar, lexis, register), skills, discourse and genres appropriate to these activities. Moreover, they listed some variable characteristics, namely that ESP may be related to or designed for specific disciplines, may use, in specific teaching situations, a different methodology from that of General English and is likely to be designed for adult learners, either at a tertiary level institution or in a professional work situation.

Some researchers tried to define ESP by means of elimination. Hutchinson and Waters (1987: 18; see Dudley-Evans – St John 1998: 25) outlined boundary conditions or baseline characteristics for ESP by stating what it is not – *not* a matter of teaching "specialised varieties" of English, *not* just a matter of science words and grammar for scientists, hotel words and grammar for hotel staff etc. and *not* different in kind from any form of language teaching, in that it should be based, in the first instance, on the principles of effective and efficient learning.

The first two claims discredit ESP pedagogy as creating field-specific vocabulary glossaries. The last statement implies that ESP practitioners should draw from what is understood as good teaching practice. In the post-method era, with the focus being on the fact that there is no single, best methodology, Hutchinson and Waters' claim that ESP is more of an approach than a product seems to have gained validity (see Dudley-Evans – St John 1998: 25). Good ESP practice should be much more than providing target language equivalents of specialised vocabulary items. It should allow the learner to function in a given, specific, often highly specialised target language situation.

More recently, Basturkmen (2006: 25) addressed the issue of ESP characteristics from a different angle, claiming that ESP can be categorized not only by domain specificity but also by the degree of learner expertise and narrow- or wide-angle course design (*Figure 1*).

Basturkmen's framework seems to be highly useful in English for Medical Purposes course design for in-service healthcare professionals, as in this case the degree of learner expertise and reasons for learning are crucial factors determining syllabus design.

*Figure 1: Categorization of ESP (after Basturkmen 2006)*

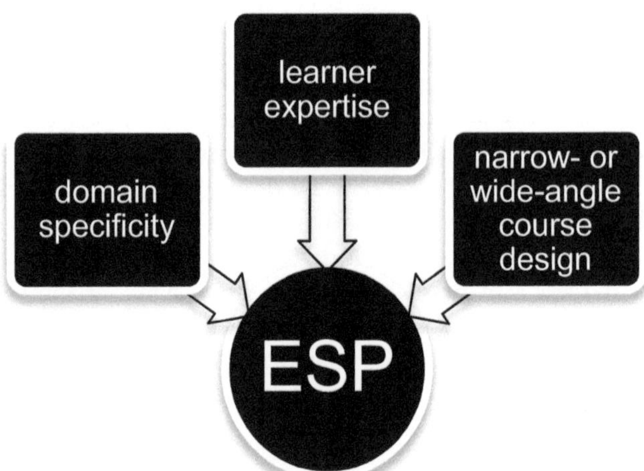


In the case of medical students, i.e. the target group researched in this book, learner expertise or, rather, the lack of it early in the undergraduate program, influences course design, transforming it into a wide-angle course. Hence, although most popular, the domain-specific categorization of ESP does not have to be the only way of classifying ESP courses. Dudley-Evans and St John (1998: 6) offer a classification based on learner experience (*Figure 2*) and make an important distinction into pre-study, in-study and post-study ESP. This is a distinction that very much holds true for teaching and learning English for Medical Purposes, as pre-study or in-study ESP methodology often has more to do with Content and Language Integrated Learning than with English for Specific Purposes, understood as language being a vehicle for communicating what one already knows. ESP courses can be defined as those where "[t]*he main element missing for the learner is how to express that conceptual knowledge he or she already has in the second language*" (Basturkmen – Elder 2004: 675), thus the goal of the course is to enable learners to use English in authentic professional situations (Antić 2010: 162).

*Figure 2: ESP classification by experience (Dudley-Evans – St John 1998, after Robinson 1991: 3–4)*

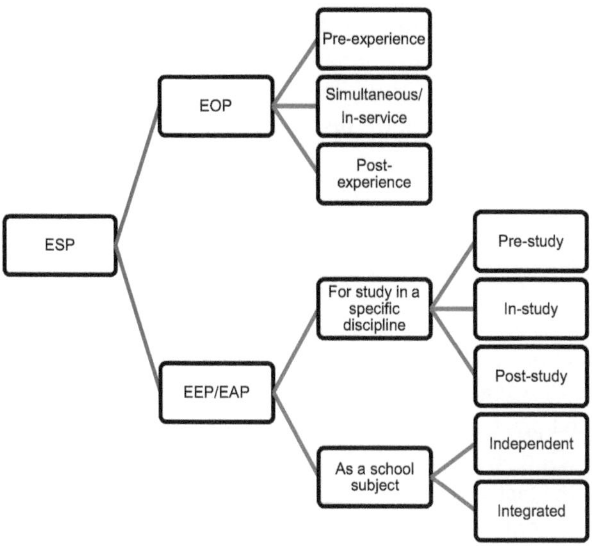


## 1.4 ESP Methodology

It is often highlighted that developments in LSP were propelled by practical rather than purely theoretical concerns (Dudley-Evans – St John 1998; Basturkmen – Elder 2004, Grucza 2013a). As good ESP practice is strongly connected to good ELT practice, throughout history two sub-fields of ESP and ELT often fed on each other – for example, in needs analysis and materials production (Dudley-Evans – St John 1998: 20).

Some researchers claim that ESP feeds on the development of English as a Lingua Franca, as many ELF publications are also relevant to ESP (Nickerson 2013: 445–446). Others highlight the role ESP played in ELT development:

> "It has been in the vanguard of the developments in ELT, moving from grammatical, functional and notional syllabuses to a more eclectic and task-based approach."
>
> (Dudley-Evans – St John 1998: 32)

What makes ESP pedagogy distinctive is the fact that the target learners already specialize in some field of study, and studying a foreign language as "a philological phenomenon" does not lie in their focus (Krickova – Polackova 2010: 221). However, it is difficult to draw a clear-cut line between ESP and EFL/ELT pedagogy as "developing an appropriate pedagogy for a specific group of learners has always been the goal of ESP practitioners" (Johns et al. 2011).

Dudley-Evans and St John (1998: I) claim the overall purpose of ESP, which is "preparing learners to communicate effectively in the task prescribed by their study or work situation," assumes an openness to drawing on research from disciplines other than applied linguistics. Therefore, ESP methodology should draw on "the methodology of the disciplines and profession it serves" (Dudley-Evans – St John 1998: 4).

Contrary to the claims by Dudley-Evans and St John (1998), for Basturkmen (2006: 5) ESP solutions seem to be indifferent to developments in SLA, and the number of publications on the effectiveness of ESP courses (Hyland 2006b), or the amount of research on learner interlanguage remains insufficient. As too little has been written on the theory of ESP learning and teaching, Basturkmen (2006: ix) makes an attempt to present a theoretical overview of the ESP field by means of drawing conclusions reaching beyond the case studies, so popular in ESP, and practical solutions adopted in particular research projects. Both observed by Dudley-Evans and St John (1998) as well as Belcher (2004), who highlighted the fact that ESP writing focused mostly on practical applications and not on theoretical frameworks.

> "Unlike other pedagogical approaches, which may be less specific needs-based and more theory-driven, ESP pedagogy places heavy demands on its practitioners to collect empirical needs-assessment data, to create or adapt materials to meet specific needs identified, and to cope with often unfamiliar subject matter and even language use…"
>
> (Belcher 2004: 166)

According to Basturkmen (2006: 3–4, after Dudley-Evans – St John 1998: 190), there are two trends in approaching ESP. It is either a genre-based approach to course development which enables to recognize *conventional formats* and prepare the course accordingly, or a deep-end strategy in which courses to a great extent rely on analysing case studies, and learners are forced to *communicate using whatever English they have at their disposal.*

Ghahremani-Ghajar et al. (2012: 269–275) criticize the fact that mainstream approaches to ESP were always instrumental – either terminology-oriented, like in register analysis (see Robinson 1980) which later developed into needs analysis and learner-oriented approaches (see Coffey 1984), or genre-based like now (see Bhatia 2004, Hyon 1996).

Basturkmen reports that, in the beginning, much of the focus in ESP was put on discovering the linguistic features of a given subject-specific language (Basturkmen 2006, after Swales 1985), e.g. the early corpus study by Barber (1966) who identified the frequency of occurrence of particular linguistic patterns, albeit, without stating the purpose for which they were used. This major flaw was resolved only in subsequent studies, which provided a correlation between the frequency of a linguistic pattern and the purpose for which it was used. Later on, identifying particular linguistic patterns became of lesser importance than developing actual learner communicative competence in a target situation (Basturkmen 2006, after Munby 1978). This change of perspective was not something unfamiliar to the whole ELT community, with the shift from structural to situational and notional-functional to communicative syllabi. According to Basturkmen in 2006, state-of-the-art ESP pedagogy focused on two elements – teaching concepts from a given discipline and, at the same time, developing the learner's linguistic/communicative competence (Basturkmen 2006). Nevertheless, as late as in 2012 Ghahremani-Ghajar et al. (2012: 269–275) complained that even within the communicative paradigm ESP is treated as a set of "fragmented components and skills" to be developed, and postulated adopting a problem-based and enquiry-based approach to ESP teaching, in which students should focus on "experiencing and challenging language in real social contexts."

Interesting as Ghahremani-Ghajar et al.'s course organisation model may sound, Basturkmen's framework seems to be more comprehensive. Basturkmen offers a framework to work one's way through ESP (Basturkmen 2006: 9) based on a triad of components: the data-driven nature of the enquiry, Structuration Theory and the framework to examine and organize work.

At this point, a word or two needs to be said about the structuration theory (Giddens 1979, 1984; in Basturkmen 2006: 10–12) which emphasizes the importance of routine and skilled performance in professional communication. Basturkmen compares this to "the rules of the game". Members of a given community, or its would-be participants, such as students of medicine, need to recognize the verbalized or unverbalized do's and don'ts, actions which are allowed or are not allowed to be performed in a particular community, and learn to play by those rules. The aim of these rules or social scripts is to facilitate conduct, i.e. action. Action is understood either as mental acts or particular social conduct. In an interesting paper, Charpy and Carnet explore the issue of acceptability and transgression within professional communities, with transgression defined as "the violation of linguistic, didactic and cultural standards accepted by the language professionals of the specialised domain" (Charpy – Carnet 2014: 7–8).

For Basturkmen, knowledge from data-driven enquiry and knowledge of the "rules of the game" are not sufficient to design and run a successful ESP course. What an ESP practitioner also needs is a framework to design and organise the work. Therefore, neither the above mentioned genre studies, nor case studies are enough to construct a fully-fledged ESP course. What is needed is a framework that would arrange all the building blocks in the most "time- and energy-efficient manner" (Basturkmen 2006: 9). Basturkmen identifies four components: Language, Learning, Teaching and Context. The Language component requires some understanding of what language is, its system and uses, hence one's definition of language heavily influences one's methods of teaching (Larsen-Freeman 2003). The Learning component involves taking into account factors such as conditions for learning and procedures used in the process of second language acquisition. The Teaching component comprises teaching methodology and course objectives. The Context component refers to the given ESP type.

The Language component and the Learning component in Basturkmen's framework correspond to Richards and Rogers' (1986) theory of the nature of language and theory of the nature of language learning, respectively (Basturkmen 2006: 13). What Basturkmen (2006: 13–14) aims at is providing ESP practitioners with some sort of a generalized tool that would make them more aware of their own approach to ESP and allow them to adopt a critical perspective. To provide an example, in a paper investigating teaching practices in the area of English for Medical Purposes in an Iranian university, Ghahremani-Ghajar et al. (2012: 269–275) recommend a contextualized and enquiry-based model of teaching English for Medical Purposes, as the idea of problem-based learning is so close to the whole idea of medical education. They suggest choosing a particular health concern, e.g. pain, as it was in their case, and arranging terminology and grammar around this problem. This way, even when students engaged in the project did not have broad medical knowledge, they were highly involved, as pain is one of the topics that everyone has experienced or has seen someone experiencing, thus the problem gained "a meaningful human context".

Another hotly debated issue in ESP is to what extent register and domain-specific discourse should influence ESP pedagogy. Many researchers claim that "(…) register cannot be used as a main basis for selection, because there is no significant way in which the language of science differs from any other kind of language" (Coffey 1984, in Hutchinson – Waters 1987: 30). However, register and discourse analysis might be helpful when considering course design. In English for Medical Purposes much depends on the vector of communication. Given the importance of doctors being able to communicate in English not only when delivering conference presentations or discussing differential diagnoses, but also "over coffee", compartmentalisation of types of English for Medical Purposes might be difficult due to its scope and versatility.

Basturkmen (2006: 27–28) makes an important distinction between things being specific and specifiable (capable of being specified), e.g. the language system is specifiable, whereas language use is specific, language skills are specifiable, but the content in which they are used is specific. Thus, when designing a course and preparing a needs analysis, it would be advisable to list the specifiables and then specify them in a given context, i.e. the EMP context. Each context would generate domain-specific problem areas, e.g. Krickova and Polackova (2010: 223) enumerate typical problems of nursing ESP in Slovakia: misspelling, false friends, use of non-existing Latin expressions or *Slenglish* – coining words that look like English words, and pronunciation.

Also, according to Flowerdew (2013: 350) there is an important choice to be made about the point of departure for genre-based teaching and learning – either *text-first* (discourse patterns) or *context-first* (content-oriented). It is frequently the case that ESP practitioners teach via metacommunicating, i.e. "the explicit analysis of examples of particular genres used in the classroom as a tool to heighten learners' awareness of genre specific features, rhetorical organization, and communicative purposes" (Flowerdew 2013: 357). As it is often argued that ESP learners benefit from this focus on genre (see Cheng 2011), the following section will provide an overview of research on genre in the field of ESP.

## 1.5 ESP Research History

The enormous expansion in science and technology led to the rise of English as a lingua franca of science. With Latin omnipresent in biomedical terminology (Ferguson 2013: 246), French and German losing their importance as languages of science in the wake of the 20th century, English remains the dominant language in the field, and researchers showed vivid interest in English for Science and Technology as early as in the 1960s (see Parkinson 2013: 155).

Although the interest in ESP can be traced back to 16th century trade and commerce, it was the 1960s that saw the development of ESP as a discipline (Dudley-Evans – St John 1998: 19). In the beginning, ESP was treated as a rather insignificant branch of English Language Teaching (Dudley-Evans – St John 1998). Grucza (2013a,b) argues convincingly that the increased importance of specific-purposes texts, caused not only the need for teaching the ability to create such texts, but also the need to educate teachers and translators. However, ESP teaching pedagogy has not received enough attention, as research in ESP started about 20–30 years ago and the Katedra Języków Specjalistycznych founded in 2000 at the University of Warsaw, was one of the first academic institutions of this kind in Europe. Nowadays, international ELT organisations such as the Teachers of English to Speakers of Other Languages Association (TESOL), the International Association of English as a Foreign Language (IATEFL) or the Association for Language Testers in Europe (ALTE) all have well-developed ESP sections (Johns – Price-Machado 2001: 52) and "action" research conducted by ESP practitioners plays an important role in refining classroom practices. Also, many institutions are interested in research into assessment in ESP and interdisciplinary course design, as well as the "language requirements of students in particular academic disciplines" (Ghahremani-Ghajar et al. 2012: 269).

Grucza (2013a) discusses the development of research in ESP in Poland, claiming that in the case of Polish research projects, the scope of research is greater as far as ESP translation is concerned, with ESP teaching methodology being underrepresented. One of the first works relating to ESP issues was Nowicki's (1978) "O ścisłość pojęć i kulturę słowa w technice", discussing the accuracy of the concepts in telecommunications and "Podstawy terminologii" (1986), where the author develops and clarifies the ideas put forward in the work from 1978 (Grucza 2013a: 20). On a more recent note, F. Grucza's "Teoretyczne podstawy terminologii" (1991) provide a comprehensive outline of terminological issues. Luckily, as the importance of ESP training programs is being acknowledged among educational institutions, there appear more and more publications on the theory of ESP learning and teaching, e.g. *LSO, FOS, Fachsprache…dydaktyka języków specjalistycznych* by Gajewska and Sowa (2014).

Following Hutchinson and Waters (1987: 9–14), ESP research went through five subsequent phases of development, or, to be precise, 4 phases by the 1980s, with the 5th phase beginning to emerge around the time they wrote the book. Hutchinson and Waters discuss the phases using the example of the development of English for Science and Technology (EST), as the most prominent branch of ESP, assuming that this illustrates the process best. The phases of ESP development identified by Hutchinson and Waters (1987) were as follows: Register Analysis, Rhetorical or Discourse Analysis, Target Situation Analysis, Skills and Strategies, A Learning-centred Approach.

These stages are also applicable to illustrate the development of interests of an ESP practitioner from an initial interest in the field, through gaining experience, to the emergence of a preferred mode of teaching. They also reflect the interest of ESP practitioners. At first, teachers who become involved in ESP usually pay attention to domain-specific vocabulary items. Then, they become more and more interested in the genre. Then, when interacting with learners, often experts in a given field, they revise their assumptions about learners' needs. To be in line with modern teaching trends, they focus on skills and strategies. Most teachers are first teachers of English and only then teachers of ESP, so the idea of skills development is familiar to them.

More recently, Johns (2013: 5–22) offers a slightly different classification of ESP research stages into: The Early Years (1962–1981), The Recent Past (1981–1990), The Modern Era (1990–2011), The Future (2011 plus). Hutchinson and Waters' stages all fall within John's *The Early Years* and *The Recent Past* category. *The Early Years* period (Johns 2013: 7–9), encompasses the time from text-based counts, i.e. *Register Analysis* in the sense of Hutchinson and Waters, and overlaps with the development of "rhetorical devices," i.e. the *Discourse Analysis* stage.

Basturkmen (2006: 69) divides ESP research according to domains of interest rather than time slots, into: Speech Acts, Genres and Social Interaction, Words with Disciplinary Specific Meanings (and structures with specific disciplinary uses).

Research into *Speech Acts* is devoted to how speakers achieve particular communicative purposes, e.g. making requests, and aims at identifying field-specific speech acts and the language structures enabling us to perform them. Research into *Genres* is devoted to the analysis of instances of field-specific key texts and "familiarizing learners" with those texts and expectations that the target-language community have about what they should contain and how they should be constructed. Research into *Social Interaction* is devoted to identifying and determining the "appropriateness" of certain linguistic devices in field-specific discourse, e.g. the use of hedges when passing on bad news in English for Medical Purposes.

Social interaction research contributes to making non-native users of field-specific discourse more sensitive to the "appropriateness" of certain forms over others, according to target culture expectations. Research into *Words with Disciplinary Specific Meanings* is often devoted to field-specific vocabulary items, such as the word "cost" in economics, and aims at identifying the most prevalent field-specific collocations so that learners are better equipped when trying to convey precise shades of meaning.

Although Basturkmen does not divide her types of research chronologically, the *Words with Disciplinary Specific Meanings* (and structures with specific disciplinary uses) research nicely fits into Hutchinson and Waters' *Register Analysis* stage. Similarly, Hutchinson and Water's stages of *Target Situation Analysis, Skills and Strategies* and *Learner-centred Stage* fall within Johns' *More Recent Past* Stage.

### 1.5.1 Register Analysis Research

The underlying assumption behind performing detailed register analysis studies was that it would enable a list of domain-specific structures and vocabulary items relevant for ESP learning and teaching to be drawn up. The concept was based on "lexicostatistics" (Dudley-Evans – St John 1998: 21, after Swales 1988) and assumed that certain forms would appear more often in ESP than in General English. Register Analysis led to the identification of key features of scientific discourse, which resulted in the development of the first research-induced ESP-tailored courses. Research conducted in the 1960s focused on grammar and lexis, e.g. Barber's (1962) study on verb forms in scientific discourse (see Johns – Price-Machado 2001: 50).

One of the earliest studies in the field of word-frequency is the corpus-based study of magazines and juvenile books by Thorndike and Lorge from 1944 (see Murray 1997: 355) which resulted in "The Teacher's Word Book of 30,000 Words". However, it was Herbert's "The Structure of Technical English" dating back to 1965 that was the first important ESP textbook (see Dudley-Evans – St John 1998: 21–22), where reading on a given topic is followed by a number of exercises dealing with sub-technical language and a given grammar point. Focus is thus placed on lexis and grammar, and not on skills development. The textbook was criticised on the grounds of, among others, passages being dense and lacking authenticity, diagrams not being supportive, exercises being repetitive and lacking in variety, as well as an extreme focus on form and a lack of focus on communication.

More or less at the same time, Higgins (1967) developed the needs and problems analysis leg of ESP. Also, Ewer and Latorre (1969) as well as Swales (1971) were trying to identify and draw up the boundaries of ESP.

One major discovery of the Register Analysis research was that, at the sentence level, the language of science was not very much different from widely used forms.

> "(…) register analysis revealed that there was very little that was distinctive in the sentence grammar of Scientific English beyond a tendency to favour particular forms (…) It did not, for example reveal any forms that were not found in General English."
>
> (Hutchinson – Waters 1987: 10)

That was grist to the mill for the part of the ELT community who never recognised ESP as anything more than being General English with some extra specific vocabulary items. What was important about early register analysis though, was that it demonstrated that General English materials might not suffice to provide a comprehensive enough range of structures characteristic of Scientific English. Register Analysis did show that certain forms were more prominent in Scientific English than in General English, which led to a shift of focus towards these forms in ESP classroom practice. For example, Harper (1986) offers a handful of conclusions drawn from an ESP programme conducted by the British Council in Saudi Arabia. Wilson (1986: 11, in Harper 1986) discusses the need to identify "systemic language" and refers to collocational analysis, as a possible solution.

Important ESP publications of the time are clearly pedagogically-oriented, e.g. "ESP at the crossroads" by Hutchinson and Waters (1980), "Further notes on developing an English programme for students of science and technology" by Ewer and Hughes-Davies (1971), "How to arm your students: A consideration of two approaches to providing materials for ESP" by Phillips and Shettlesworth (1978), "Writing Scientific English" by Swales (1971), or "Nucleus General Science" by Dudley-Evans and Bates. Also, Lackstrom, Selinker and Trimble's "Grammar and Technical English" (1972), and Tarone, Dwyer, Gillette and Icke's "On the use of the passive in astrophysics papers" (1981) are often referred to as publications that set the academic standards at the time (Johns et al. 2011: 2).

Collocation analysis, paired with expert knowledge in a given field was often used to specify which forms should be given extra attention. Wilson (1986, in Harper 1986) sees collocation analysis as a means of maximizing the efficiency of a language learning programme, with the focus being placed on written scientific language as being easier to examine. However, she does not discard the possibility of a collocational analysis of spoken language. In a similar vein, as early as in 1981, Tarone et al. investigated the occurrence of the passive voice in astrophysics. More recently, Pinto dos Santos (2002, in Basturkmen – Elder 2004: 675) performed an analysis of the correspondence between pharmaceutical companies, and the results of the study served as a basis to develop instructional materials.

Soler (2002, in Basturkmen – Elder 2004: 675) conducted research focusing on the use of adjectives in biochemistry texts, and then suggested ways to improve article writing among university students. Ferguson (2001, in Basturkmen – Elder 2004: 675 and Ferguson 2013) examined the use of if-conditionals in medical writing. Lindemann and Mauranen (2001, in Basturkmen 2006) investigated the occurrence of the word "just" in academic discourse.

Currently, corpora are often used to assess concordance at sentence level or determine the most common lexical collocations (Johns – Price-Machado 2001: 51), e.g. Sullivan and Girginer (2002, in Basturkmen – Elder 2004: 674) compiled a corpus of pilot and air traffic controllers' language in Turkey from spoken data obtained at the airport.

Cook (2003: 73) lends support to the question of the significance of collocational language, and enumerates two areas of SLA research as especially promising: corpus linguistics and research into collocations, as helpful in recognizing "patterns and regularities of language use," as well as "frequent combinations of words". With regards to the correlation between the use of corpora and collocational language, Cook makes claims for their relevance to language teaching pedagogy:

> "As records of language behaviour, corpora cannot tell us directly how language is represented in the mind. The fact that something occurs frequently in a corpus does not necessarily mean that it is processed as a ready-made unit by each individual user. Nevertheless, the prominence of collocation does strongly suggest a greater role for memory in language processing than was previously thought. Language processing may be less a question of slotting individual words into a grammatical structure and far more a question of deploying larger units made up of several words."
>
> Cook (2003: 73–74)

For example, based on a corpus study of temporal conjunctions used by native and Taiwanese physicians in medical case presentations, Hung et al. conclude that "general English grammatical writing instruction may not be effective for non-native physicians who need to pay more attention to chronological writing in order to conduct precise medical writing" (Hung et al. 2010: 263–265).

To conclude, attractive as register analysis may have seemed at first sight, it did not support the idea that domain-specific language would be a clearly distinctive variety of English, using forms that would not be encountered in communication in English for General Purposes (Hutchinson – Waters 1987: 31). At this point, it is important to highlight that the main focus of register analysis was on sentence level forms, which turned out to be a serious limitation to this approach. Nor did register analysis answer the question why certain forms were used more frequently than others (Dudley-Evans – St John 1998: 22).

### 1.5.2 Rhetorical or Discourse Analysis Research

With sentence-level register analysis having been dismissed as insufficient to provide the answers, the discourse analysis approach took over in accounting for the lack of ultimate success in ESP learners. One of the key tenets of this stage in ESP methodology development was coming to realize that the problem lay in the ineffectiveness of an ESP learner in performing "a communicative act" in the target language context/situation, and not in their inability to produce an acceptable English sentence. Thus, the sentence-level syllabus course structure was replaced by a syllabus structure organised around some text organisational patterns, such as making a recommendation, stating purpose or expressing causality.

The pattern-recognition approach was implemented in teaching practice, e.g. in the form of publications such as "English for Science and Technology: A Discourse Approach" (Richards 1976), or "Grammar and Technical English" (Lackstrom et al. 1972) which developed the idea of relating language form to language use (Dudley-Evans – St John 1998: 22). The Washington School research group led by Larry Selinker, Louis P. Trible and John Lackstrom (Johns 2013: 7–8) described rhetorical considerations regarding context for sentence use.

> "From the mid-1970s into the 1980s the focus switched more and more to spoken interactions based first on a grammatical, and then gradually more functional, construct. Materials were based in functions such as Greetings, Making Introductions, Making Arrangements, Agreeing and Disagreeing. Formulaic language and gambits were taught and practised in dialogues and role plays."
>
> (Dudley-Evans – St John 1998: 29)

To illustrate this tendency, Hutchinson and Waters (1987: 29) provide an example of two technical texts of the same illocutionary force but differing to a great extent. One of the texts is a transcript of a video-taped instruction, the other is an instruction taken from a manual. Register analysis and discourse analysis of these two texts show these are two very different texts and two very different communication situations. Thus, the needs of communicators involved in these acts are different.

Basturkmen (2006: 47) highlights the fact that ESP is vividly interested in how particular functions are expressed by members of a given ESP community and there is evidence showing that non-native speakers tend to use different speech acts to perform the same functions than those native speakers would use in the same situation (Basturkmen 2006: 50). Basturkmen refers to research by Bardovi-Harlig (2001, in Basturkmen 2006: 50–51) identifying possible differences, regardless of the level of non-native speakers' grammatical competence, in the choice of speech acts themselves – for example, native speakers were more likely to use constructions expressing suggestions and non-native speakers were more likely to use more forms expressing obligation. The forms chosen by non-native speakers were perceived as less natural in a given situation. As genre is a reflection of how things are done by a given community, for Paltridge (2000, in Basturkmen 2006: 59) it is not enough for learners to master the formula used in a given genre, but they also need to understand and grasp the feeling of why, and for what reason such constructions are used. This might be an explanation to why natives use more suggestions and non-natives more rejection phrases. Here comes the role of the ESP teacher, whose job is to make learners more sensitive to the subtleties of a specific genre. Teaching formulaic expressions is not enough. Just as in Larsen-Freeman's approach (2003) one needs to teach the form, meaning but also context in which it is used, and if necessary raise the learner's awareness of the subtleties so that they can fit better the community they wish to be a part of. Basturkmen (2006: 62) gives an example from English for Medical Purposes, where it might be beneficial for the teacher to explain the use of hedges in doctor-patient communication, especially when passing on bad news, so that non-native doctors do not sound indifferent, or even rude.

### 1.5.3 The Recent Past Research

According to Johns (2013: 9–12), 1981 and the publication of "Aspects of Article Introductions" by Swales as well as the concept of rhetorical moves, marked another chapter in the history of ESP. Prior to that, researchers focused on text analysis and many did not bother to consult experts in the field (Johns 2013: 8). It was only around 1981 that the opinion of experts in a given discipline was taken into account, for example, in "The language of science from the viewpoint of the writer of science" (Godman 1976).

Some of the more important works of the time regarding English for Medical Purposes include: "Medical discourse: Aspects of author's comment" by Adams Smith (1984), "The development of English as the international language of medicine" by Maher (1986), "Tests as knowledge claims: The social construction of two biologists' articles" by Myers (1985*)* or on a psychological note "Studies of Doctor-Patient interaction" by Roter and Hall (1989). Also, Malcolm's (1987, see Johns 2013: 10) "What rules govern tense usage in scientific articles?" Betty Lou DuBois was one of the more prolific authors in the area of biomedical writing, with publications on "The Use of Slides in Biomedical Speeches" (1980), "The Construction of Noun Phrases in Biomedical Journal Articles" (1981), "Paragraph Structure of Biomedical Speeches: Preliminary Report" (1983) or the design and presentation of biomedical posters ("Poster Sessions at Biomedical Meetings: Design and Presentation", 1985). Important works written in the 1990s include: "Hedges and Textual Communicative Function in Medical English Written Discourse" by Salager-Meyer (1994), "The representation of truth in academic medical writing" by Skelton (1997) or, on a psychological note, "Doctor-Patient Communication a Review of Literature" by Ong et al. (1995).

The end of the Recent Past category was marked by the appearance of "Genre Analysis" (Swales 1990). Its final stage was also delineated by the appearance of "English for Specific Purposes. A Learning-centred Approach" (Hutchinson – Waters 1987). In 1993, Bhatia published "Analysing Genre: Language Use in Professional Settings" in which he offers pedagogical implications in a seven-step model:

- placing the given genre-text in a situational context,
- surveying existing literature,
- refining the situational/contextual analysis,
- selecting corpus,
- studying the institutional context,
- levels of linguistic analysis: analysis of lexico-grammatical features; analysis of text-patterning or textualization; structural interpretation of the text genre,
- specialist information in genre analysis.

Genre analysis aimed at explaining why a particular genre-text is written the way it is, and it was an attempt to provide a framework for ESP practitioners and non-native ESP users to find their way around ESP rhetorics. However, following Cook (2003: 75) even detailed analysis of factual linguistic information was not a sufficient predictor of success in learning English for Specific Purposes, hence the shift towards target situation analysis.

### 1.5.4 Target Situation Analysis (Needs Analysis)

Currently, there is nothing particularly insightful in claiming that a detailed needs analysis is conducive to good teaching practice. Belcher (2009b: 3, in Paltridge – Starfield 2013: 6) highlights the responsibility on the part of the ESP professionals to find out what the learners need to be familiar with to be successful. However, this was not always the case. At first it was the teacher's intuition that determined what should be taught, only then did it turn into target situation analysis (Flowerdew 2013: 326–328). The 1970s saw a growth in interest in needs analysis as due to the necessity for ESP learners to perform "communicative acts" in the target language context. Identifying the situations involving communication became the nub of the matter for ESP researchers. Thus Needs Analysis or Target Situation Analysis (as Hutchinson and Waters choose to call it after Chambers 1980) became a prominent field of inquiry in ESP methodology.

> "What distinguishes ESP from General English is not the existence of a need as such but rather an awareness of the need."
>
> (Hutchinson – Waters 1987: 53)

Target Situation Analysis was an important step in the attempts to arrive at "a workable definition of ESP" (Hutchinson – Waters 1987: 3). Flowerdew (2013: 325) gives a definition of needs analysis by Hyland (2006a: 73) as focusing on relevant and effective course design based on information about the participants. Thus, the "what" of the course should encompass "what learners know, don't know or want to know."

The mushrooming Target Situation Analysis based ESP courses related to the learner's target language "necessities", "lacks" and "wants" (Hutchinson – Waters 1987: 55–56), taking into consideration the fact that there might be a conflict between what the learners think their necessities are and what course designers think their necessities are, as this issue can be quite contentious in ESP. What is more, the position of the ESP learner as an expert in the field, results in his stronger position in the classroom. With background expert knowledge in L1, learners have more authority to decide what is of use to them and what is not. Contrary to the two previous stages of ESP development, the main focus of the Needs Analysis Stage was on the learner rather than on the language itself.

Johns and Price-Machado (2001: 43) highlight the fact that the needs of ESP learners are easier to identify due to the clear professional or occupational setting. Also, the learners being adults, one should assume adult-proper methodology. Together with developments in ELT at the time, this was moving away from the claim that register analysis of ESP texts combined with a structural syllabus might actually do the trick.

According to Hutchinson and Waters (1987: 12), initially, it seemed that the communicative angle that had been adapted in ESP allowed it to become a successful comprehensive, fully-fledged, systematised, learner-centred teaching approach. However, it soon revealed its shortcomings. Hutchinson and Waters discuss the failure of Munby's (1978, in Hutchinson – Waters 1987: 54) Communication Needs Processor, used to identify target language needs, claiming that it demonstrated how little can be learned from performing such an analysis. One of the more popular models was that of Munby's (1978, in Dudley-Evans – St John 1998: 25), but it was criticized on the grounds that it did not specify which language forms correlated with which needs. Dudley-Evans and St John claimed that Munby's model was too complex to have a significant influence on actual ESP practice, but was a landmark in the field of ESP. It was a sign of the field maturing.

Basturkmen (2006: 18–20) assumes a critical approach towards the numerous needs analysis studies available in the literature, claiming that they have major flaws, e.g. it is often the institutions that decide upon what the students require, while learners often do not realize what their needs are, there is little differentiation between objective needs and subjective needs, or that very often language needs are not the same as learning needs. Basturkmen (2006: 28) claims it is rarely the case that needs analysis is unbiased and objective. She argues that it is often influenced by institutional demands and underestimates the subjective needs of learners.

If we treat language as a tool, and learning ESP is rarely learning English for the sake of learning the English language system, but rather a vehicle that enables functioning in a particular workplace environment (Basturkmen 2006: 18), then we should probably adopt some sort of task-based approach in which we focus on achieving maximum "linguistic efficiency" within particular time constraints (West 1994, in Basturkmen 2006: 18). In examining the parameters of linguistic efficiency in a given time constraint, ESP practitioners need to discriminate between what can or cannot be done during a particular course (Basturkmen 2006: 23). Obviously, teaching "all of the language" is out of the question for practical reasons. A detailed needs analysis should help us to make a proper choice of objectives, which is in line with Johns and Price-Machado's (2001: 49) claim that needs assessment is an indispensable prerequisite of "genuine" ESP practice.

As far as Target Needs Analysis in English for Medical Purposes is concerned, one of the first analyses available is Allwright and Allwright's (1977) needs analysis, which allowed them to establish twelve situations of potential difficulty that non-native doctors might encounter (Allwright and Allwritght 1977: 58, in Ferguson 2013: 255). The situations were as follows:

- Rapid reading of textbooks/professional journals/papers for information,
- Detailed study of textbooks/journals/papers etc.
- Writing papers/reports/articles in English for publications/symposia/conferences,
- Corresponding with English-speaking colleagues on professional matters,

- Understanding lectures/papers in English delivered orally at conferences, medical meetings, symposia etc.
- Giving papers/lectures in English at conferences, medical meetings, symposia etc.
- Participating in (i.e. understanding and contributing to) formal discussion at conferences, etc.
- Participating in (i.e. understanding and contributing to) informal discussion at conferences, etc.
- Participating in post-graduate courses in English speaking medical institutions,
- Entertaining/being entertained,
- Doing clinical work with English-speaking patients,
- Doing clinical work with English-speaking colleagues.

At this point, it is important to highlight that, contrary to healthcare practitioners, students of medicine, being at the beginning of their careers in the field, might not, and usually are not, aware of their linguistic needs as far as English for Medical Purposes is concerned (see Antić 2010: 159). However, they do realize that "[a] good knowledge of general and medical English is a prerequisite for professional improvement and progress" (Antić 2010: 160).

> "In these cases the courses aim to help the learners become better equipped linguistically to cope with the communicative demands they face in their work or study situations."
>
> (Basturkmen – Elder 2004: 673)

Currently, the tendency is to engage learners in "occluded genres", e.g. nursing care plans (Belcher 2013: 542, Shi 2009, Hussin 2004). Also, there is much interest in professional – non-professional communication. For example, a study by Bosher and Smalkowski (2002, in Basturkmen – Elder 2004: 674), revealed that what constituted the biggest problem for non-English-speaking students in a nursing programme was communicating in clinical settings, not only with patients but also with colleagues.

Nonetheless, needs-sensitive, synthetic syllabi, organized around notional-functional skills were based on the intuitions of applied linguists and language teachers to a greater extent than they should and experts were not involved in the process enough (Long 2005, in Flowerdew 2013: 328). Consequently, as Long suggests, task-based needs analysis is "a more reliable source of data than those produced by language teachers and applied linguists" (Flowerdew 2013: 328). Long's needs analysis incorporated both inductive and deductive procedures. Flowerdew (2013) highlights the importance of inductive procedures:

> "As the ESP teacher is more often than not the "non-knower," unstructured interviews with domain specialists would seem a good method to use initially for deriving categories for follow-up survey questionnaires or structured interviews."
>
> (Flowerdew 2013: 330)

Antić, on the other hand, (2010: 159–163) highlights the importance of deductive methods of needs analysis, when describing a study in which student errors were analyzed and served as a working basis for improvements in course design.

Basturkmen (2010: 143, in Flowerdew 2013: 330) offers an interesting model of course design in which the course specification emerges from data analysis combined with pedagogical descriptions, which, on the other hand, emerge from initial needs analysis and involve: 1) Level 1 – below surface analysing needs 2) Level 2 – below surface investigating discourse and 3) Level 3 – above surface determining the curriculum.

### 1.5.5 Towards the New

Interest in this field of ESP research was what might plausibly be argued as the first attempt to analyze not just the surface forms of ESP but also the underlying skills and strategies. This approach drew inspiration from developments in the field of cognitive science. Learning and teaching was supposed to be meaning- and not form-driven. The mental makeup of an ESP text was more important than its surface form and the aim of ESP was to enable the learner to extract meaning from a given type of domain-specific text, with focus often being placed on reading and listening strategies. This approach is still clearly visible in the attitudes of experts towards scientific texts. More often than not, what is important for them is the actual meaning, whereas how it is passed on is of lesser importance.

However, some researchers claim that, contrary to other types of ESP where one specific language skill is often favoured, in the case of English for Medical Purposes all skills are equally important and the context requires that they all be practiced equally (Antić 2010: 162). Following Basturkmen (2006: 25, after Long – Crooks 1992), it is claimed that ESP tasks are determined by their relevance to real world events in the target environments. In the case of EMP these would include, e.g. simulated case conferences, listen and report tasks, read and report tasks, listening to a talk from a guest speaker doctor, preparing and presenting short talks, acting out doctor-patient role-plays or tasks involving medical English pronunciation practice with the use of authentic texts and prioritization of listening and speaking (Ferguson 2013: 256–257).

The new generation of publications currently used in ESP practice, e.g. "100 Cases in Clinical Medicine" by Rees et al. (2007), "English in Medicine" by Gledinning and Holmström (2005) or "Professional English in Use: Medicine" by Gledinning and Howard (2007), to mention just a few, place considerable attention to practicing skills, however, sometimes to the detriment of the range of lexis available.

Hutchinson and Waters' investigation of ESP teaching practice lent support to the claim that even the most accurate description of a given genre does not directly result in language learning. Although the question of "what" to teach still remains valid, to some researchers a far more important question than the method of teaching (Salager 1983: 62), what ESP practice requires is a learning-centred model (see Hutchinson – Waters 1987: 49–50) consisting of carefully planned communication tasks.

John's Modern Era period starts around 1990 and is marked by the appearance of two ESP journals (Johns 2013: 13): *Journal of Second Language Writing* (JSLW) in 1991 by Ilona Leki and Tony Silva and *Journal of English for Academic Purposes* (JEAP) in 2001 by Liz Hamp-Lyons and Ken Hyland. This stage is also marked by increased interest in corpus-based research and a surge in the number of publications concerning the intercultural aspects of ESP, so-called "intercultural rhetorics" (see Connor 2002, 2004, in Johns 2013: 13). It was also in the 1990s that it became popular to publish in international journals to boost university rankings (Johns 2013: 13).

The drive for convergence of ESP theory, research and pedagogical practice (see the discussion in Johns 2013: 14) gave rise to many interesting publications, e.g. "Genre Analysis: English in Academic and Research Settings" by John M. Swales (1990). Other interesting studies were conducted by Salager-Meyer (1992) on verb tense and modality in medical English abstracts, Lores (2004) on research article abstracts, Kanoksilapathan (2007) on the language of biochemistry articles, Gotti and Salager (2006) on advances in medical English discourse analysis, Salager-Meyer et al. (2013) on titling and authorship practices in medical case reports, or Salager-Meyer et al. (2010) on a cross-linguistic/cultural analysis of acknowledgments in medical research papers.

The scope of English as the language of science seems to be expanding. Parkinson (2013, after Halliday 1993) presents the expanding focus of EST, from the innermost linguistic perspective to the outermost cultural perspective. As a vehicle used to pass on certain information, English does more than get a message across, it also influences disciplinary socialization and discipline-specific culture and values.

*Figure 3: The expanding focus of EST (Parkinson 2013, after Halliday 1993)*

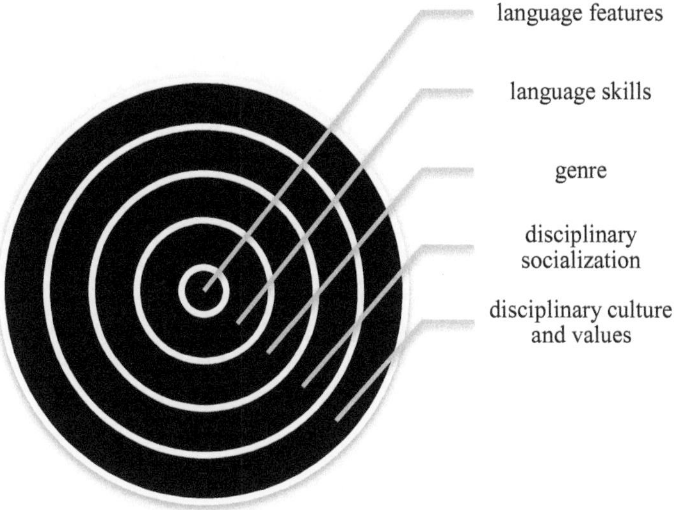


As outlined on the preceding pages, ESP research has more often than not dealt with English as the language of science and technology, e.g. a study by Mudraya (2006) on the use of collocations to distinguish between a general and a special meaning of a word. Parkinson (2013: 164–168) discusses important features of English for Science and Technology such as nominalizations or impersonal style recalling a study by Mohan and Beckett (2003) on nominalizations in teacher talk. The study demonstrated that teachers were likely to recast students to sound more nominalised, and nominalizations are preferred over clausal packaging of meaning, as they allow for a more efficient use of the theme-rheme pattern of sentences, and thus more effective presentation of cause-effect sequences. Johns (2013: 19) highlights the importance of collaboration between ESP practitioners, corpora researchers and, importantly, employers, so that students learn relevant things. John's *The Future period* is marked by such publications as "New Directions in English for Specific Purposes Research" by Diane Belcher, Ann M. Johns and Brian Paltridge (2011) who argue that for ESP to be successful, learner identity and culture need to be given more prominence, or the collection of papers on the interplay of the language and the content knowledge components among non-native medical practitioners "English Language and the Medical Profession: Instructing and Assessing the Communication Skills of International Physicians" by edited by Barbara J. Hoekje and Sara M. Tipton (2011).

## 1.6 Concluding Remarks

This chapter has examined the theoretical background related to the core assumptions about English for Specific Purposes. Given the vast scope of the field in question, an attempt was made to provide an overview of developments in ESP research from its beginnings to the present. It can be concluded that the importance of English for Specific Purposes lies not only in its function as a "vehicle" for communication, but also as an integrating factor in professional communities allowing their members to benefit from accumulated knowledge (see the discussion in Grucza 2013b: 6–12). The field of ESP methodology grapples with its problems (see the discussion in Arabski 2002, Grucza 2013a, 2013b). Nonetheless, it needs to be highlighted at this point that the growing interest in English for Specific Purposes ought to pave the way for more action research devoted to ESP teaching pedagogy.

# Chapter Two: Key Features of English for Medical Purposes

## 2.1 Introduction

Being able to write and communicate in English has become an important predictor of a healthcare professional's career (see the discussion in Basturkmen 2006, Ferguson 2013, Flowerdew 2013, Krickova – Polackova 2010, Parkinson 2000, Ribes et al. 2010, Taylor 2005, among others). English is undeniably "the lingua franca of medical studies and practice and (...) the command of English has become a key pre-requisite for doing clinical or theoretical research and taking part in international biomedical communication" (Charpy – Carnet 2014: 4). Being a member of a discourse community involves using its characteristic language and genres, and also sharing its values (which are reflected in its language and genres), and taking on a role recognized by other members of the discourse community (Paltridge 2012, in Parkinson 2013: 156).

It is often the case that the professional success of researchers depends on their ability to publish a paper in prestigious journals. Taylor (2005: 3) quotes a study conducted at Johns Hopkins Medical School which revealed that the number of published articles directly correlated with the likelihood of being promoted. This study was conducted in 1988, but nowadays, the "publish or perish" tendency causes even greater rise in the number of international submissions for SSCI journals, which, presumably, makes the correlation even stronger. Johns (2013: 13) highlights the importance of academics publishing in international journals to boost university rankings. Non-native authors may be at a disadvantage as far as the possibility of getting published is concerned (Antić et al. 2013, Ferguson 2013: 246, Carli – Ammon 2007, Benfield – Howard 2000, Benfield – Feak 2006). Perhaps, Institutes of English studies should recognize the importance of scientific writing as a branch of academic writing and offer more courses of that sort. Many students of English studies pursue their careers in publishing houses, and more and more people are faced with the need to be able to proofread or edit an article in scientific English, whereas research writing and reading are underrepresented in teaching materials. On the one hand, many publications of non-native authors resemble sentences glued up from different articles in a given field of study, to an extent we might find difficult to accept on grounds of plagiarism. On the other hand, there seems to be a finite number of ways one can present statistical data or describe a medical case. What is more, scientific journals strive for uniformity by providing detailed guidelines for authors, or through the necessity of using the IMRD format.

As there is a growing demand for doctors to deliver conference presentations and papers in English, as well as to be able to communicate with English speaking patients, not surprisingly, there is exponential interest in efficient teaching and learning of English for Medical Purposes at university level (Antić 2010, 2014; Coxhead 2013; Ribes et al. 2010; Rogers 2007; Taylor 2005; Wang et al. 2008). Also, there emerged a "need to develop a widely-accepted proficiency test for healthcare professionals taking into account these discursive and cultural variations within the context of a communicative approach" (Charpy – Carnet 2014: 4).

## 2.2 Core Features of English for Medical Purposes

English for Medical Purposes is an "umbrella" term, all depending on the vector of communication. Following Charpy and Carnet (2014: 4) "(…) communication between senior doctors, junior doctors, medical students and patients may fluctuate from EMP to English for General Purposes (EGP) with popularisation in between." Given the importance of being able to communicate in English, not only in professional situations but also "over coffee", a comprehensive compartmentalisation of types of EMP might be difficult, due to its scope and versatility.

Broadly speaking, there are many types of sources we can refer to, trying to define the scope of English for Medical Purposes (e.g. Ribes et al. 2010: ix):

- Scientific writing: articles, journals, textbooks, abstracts, letters of referral, clinical studies protocols, informed consent forms, surgical protocols;
- Spoken language: conference presentations, doctor-patient language, domain specific jargon, being on duty, differential diagnoses, discussing test results;
- Sub-scientific writing: publications/websites aimed at non-qualified readers, films or videos;
- Corpora;
- Language used in hospital-based films or series.

Ferguson makes a distinction in teaching related EMP literature. Although he admits that these categories cannot be entirely made separate, Ferguson (2013: 243) makes an attempt to distinguish two types of texts:

- "literature of particular relevance to English for medical purposes (EMP), a pedagogic and research enterprise focusing on improving the English language skills of non-Anglophone health professionals"

- "literature on health care communication, and especially doctor-patient communication."

Ferguson highlights the fact that health communication is a widely researched topic with implications having a direct impact on the improvement of the quality and effectiveness of clinical practice. The findings of health communication research find their way into textbooks and publications aimed at non-native users of English for medical purposes. These two branches of literature seem to be feeding on each other in a feedback mechanism. Current research findings on health communication are transferred to EMP coursebooks and courses. New generations of professionals are being trained according to modernised guidelines and standards in clinical practice.

The distinction into "health professionals talking to other health professionals" English and "health professionals talking to patients" English brings about a number of decisions to be made when designing an EMP course. From my experience, the latter is more difficult for non-native learners of EMP in a foreign language classroom setting due to the lack of knowledge about colloquial equivalents of medical terms. Doctor-Patient English is an important component of modern, communicatively-oriented textbooks for health professionals, as when talking to other doctors, health professionals can to a great extent rely on "common core knowledge" and Latinate terms.

### 2.2.1 Impact of Latin on Medical Terminology

It is widely known that Latin and Latinized Greek constitute the core of medical terminology (Taylor 2005: 49–50). For many centuries, Latin played the role of the language of science, enabling concepts to be labelled in a unified way. However, the developments in the field of medicine brought about the necessity to expand the existing lexicon. Latin turned out to be unable to accommodate these developments and as a result, there appeared more and more medical terms of English origin.

Džuganová (2013: 55) distinguishes two trends in medical terminology: precisely worked-out and internationally standardised anatomical nomenclature, and the rapidly developing non-standardised terminologies of individual clinical branches. While many Latin and Greek terms were built by derivation, e.g. myocardium (myo+card[ium]), endocarditis (endo+card+itis), terms which are not Latinate in origin are often formed by means of compounding, e.g. blood donor, hay fever, Black Death, sleepwalker, life-span, collar-bone, birth-control, gallstone (Džuganová 2013: 58). And nowadays, the most common way of forming medical terms is neither derivation nor compounding, but syntactic (i.e. forming multi-word phrases), e.g. AIDS Acquired Immune Deficiency Syndrome, SARS Severe Acute Respiratory Syndrome or IBS Irritable Bowel Syndrome (Džuganová 2013: 58–59). These terms are then very often used only in abbreviated form, e.g. GP (General Practitioner), or as acronyms or initialisms, e.g. DNA for deoxyribonucleic acid. ROHHAD syndrome (Rapid-onset Obesity with Hypothalamic dysfunction, Hypoventilation and Autonomic Dysregulation) can serve as one more example of that sort, as this term functions as a proper noun, e.g. children with ROHHAD. Backronyms are also frequently used in medical terminology. Džuganová (2013: 67) gives an interesting example of the Apgar score. The commonly known rating system for newborns was developed by Virginia Apgar, and then for educational reasons, a backronym was devised to reflect the scoring criteria (Appearance, Pulse, Grimace, Activity, Respiration). Džuganová (2013: 59–60) also mentions marginal types of forming medical terms, such as conversion, i.e. verbs developing from nouns – e.g. position – to position; back-formation, i.e. creating a new lexeme by removing affixes – e.g. euthanase from euthanasia, syringe from syringes (Latin: syrinx); clipping, i.e. dropping part of the word – e.g. polio(myelitis), doc(tor), flu(influenza). Also, many loanwords and borrowings (Džuganová 2013: 61–62) have found their way into medical English: from French – e.g. bowel, curette, denture, diarrhoea, malaise; from Latin – e.g. femur, humerus, mandible, puncture, pulp; of Germanic origin – e.g. hand, finger, nose, arm, chin; from Greek – e.g. diabetes, emphysema, myopia, pneumonia, trauma. Another interesting feature of Medical English is the fact that there exist a number of Greek or Latin terms emerging at the same time (Džuganová 2013: 61–62):

*Table 1: Variation in medical terminology (after Džuganová 2013)*

| **Two Greek/Latin terms emerging at the same time** | | |
|---|---|---|
| antiaemophylic factor A | & | coagulation factor |
| asiderotic anaemia | & | sederopenic anaemia |
| heamatopoiesis | & | sanguinification |
| erythrocyte | & | normocyte |
| **Translation of a Greek/Latin term** | | |
| erythrocyte | & | red blood cell (RBC) |
| leukocyte | & | white blood cell (WBC) |
| thrombocyte | & | blood platelet |
| coagulation | & | blood clotting |
| haemolysis | & | blood destruction |
| heamostatis | & | arrest of bleeding |

| Variations of a translation of a term |
|---|
| Phagocyte/phagocytic cell/defensive cell |
| Hodgkin's disease/Hodgkin's granuloma/Hodgkin's sarcoma |

Ribes et al. (2010) provide an extensive list of Latin based medical vocabulary items, among which there are many irregular plurals. However, from a teaching point of view, Latin or Greek based terms are not much of a problem, as students of medicine attending lectures have a good command of those anyway. The most important, troublesome things about them is their correct pronunciation. What poses a greater challenge to non-Anglophone healthcare practitioners are colloquial equivalents, eponyms, culture specific toponyms or clippings used in spoken medical jargon for the sake of economizing and effectiveness. And although medical terminology is being unified in the form of ICD (International Classification of Diseases) the process concerns mostly technical terms, while colloquial names or emerging specialized terms are more of a problem.

## 2.2.2 Core Lexical Features of EMP

Many researchers have attempted to characterise medical English for descriptive or practical reasons. Ferguson (2013: 252) discusses research related to the grammatical features of medical writing, claiming that most studies would embrace the lexico-grammar bond. The perspective on ESP vocabulary illustrates the overall opposing tendencies in defining ESP which have been discussed earlier in this work. It either deals with a common core and then expands it to specialised items, or treats all language as language for specific purposes (Coxhead 2013: 116, after Basturkmen 2006).

In its initial stages, ESP research analysis focused on corpus lexicostatistics (Swales 1985, in Basturkmen 2006: 63–66), i.e. determining field-specific lexical items and most frequent items in field-specific structures, with an assumption that some lexical items would appear more often than others. The fascination with concordancing software revealed differences in certain words in General English and in English for Medicine. Basturkmen (2006: 63–66) gives an example of the word *present* used more often as a noun in General English and more often as a verb in Medical English, e.g. *She presented with severe weight loss; The patients presented with pain in the upper right molar*. Showing that *present with* is a field-specific structure that would not be as frequently encountered in General English is important from a pedagogical viewpoint.

In search of establishing a "core" medical lexis, Salager (1983) performed a statistical analysis of 100,000 medical words regardless of the medical specialization. His research had some pedagogical implications. Although Salager's study focused mostly on reading comprehension, his observations led him to conclude that the detailed analysis of a medical corpus allows the quality of ESP courses to be improved. Salager referred to earlier studies in the field (Edwards 1974, Martin 1976, Anderson 1980, Hoffman 1981, Pica 1981, Qvistgaard 1981) which pointed to the fact that there is a certain group of vocabulary items which might pose a serious obstacle to non-native readers of medical texts. Salager discusses early frequency lists by Greenhall (1981) and Qvistgaard (Salager 1983: 55) as an inspiration for his corpus study. In his corpus, which was made up of 100,000 items from 50 texts in 12 specialisations (from textbooks or journals), Salager performed a frequency count and divided the words in the corpus into 3 groups (Salager 1983: 56–57):

- Basic English (BE) – part of the lexicon common to all kinds of writing, whether it be scientific, technical or literary;
- Fundamental Medical English (FME) – made up of those roots whose frequency of occurrence is homogeneously distributed over the whole corpus but in a significantly different way than in BE,
- Specialized Medical English (SME) – composed of specialized terms particular to a given discipline and known only to the small group of workers in that field.

Salager found 1,425 roots of statistical significance to the study. He compares the results of his earlier study from 1977 on engineering and Osuna's study on biology (1982) to conclude that the percentages of roots forming each stratum are very similar (Salager 1983: 57) in these studies, and the difference doesn't demonstrate statistical significance ($p<0.05$). Obviously, Salager's study, or any corpus based study, involves a lot of arbitrary decision-making, which might constitute a big disadvantage of these projects. What is more, taking into account the developments in medicine since the 1960s, we might assume that Salager's list would be of little value to modern ESP teaching. Nevertheless, as has already been mentioned, early research on medical corpora laid the foundations of modern EMP teaching.

More recently, Ferguson (2013: 253) quotes a study by Chung and Nation (2003), who discovered that technical words in anatomy texts constituted as much as 37.6 percent of word types, whereas in applied linguistics texts, for example, technical words only accounted for 16.3 percent. Therefore, it comes as no surprise that the learning and teaching of English for Medical Purposes is most often associated with learning terminological equivalents. Another point made by Ferguson is that core medical terminology is only one type of item to be taught. Semi-technical vocabulary, or academic medical vocabulary seem to be of great importance as well, as far as course development or materials development are concerned. Also Coxhead (2013: 115–132) makes an attempt to define the scope of specific vocabulary in English for Specific Purposes, as even after so many years of research, the scope of the specialized vocabulary lexicon has not been determined (Coxhead 2013: 116). Available estimates, e.g. by Nation (2008: 10, in Coxhead 2013: 116) showing that technical vocabulary might range from 1,000 to 5,000 words are far from satisfactory. Coxhead makes a point, saying that specialized vocabulary does not necessarily have to mean Greco-Latin words or highly technical words (Coxhead 2013: 116), it is rather a matter of the range of meanings of a given item, e.g. *by-pass* in medical English (Nation 2008). Following Coxhead (2013: 127), one of the problems encountered by ESP practitioners might be to identify everyday words that take on a particular meaning in a specialized context, e.g. *dissolve* becomes a technical word in chemistry or biology. What is more, with the developments in the field, there frequently appear new terms, or old terms acquire a new meaning (Crawford Camiciottoli 2007: 138, in Coxhead 2013: 128). However, identifying these vocabulary items is one thing, and using them in the classroom is another. Compiling a corpus is one thing, but being able to make use of it in foreign language teaching is another. Coxhead (2013: 129, in Byrd – Coxhead 2010) makes a strong claim that ESP practitioners lack information on the use of target words and bundles.

Coxhead (2013: 116) gives a number of reasons why vocabulary is important in ESP, e.g. both teachers and learners wish to teach/learn relevant items, and domain-specific terminology gives them a sense of not wasting their time. What's more, learning the jargon makes learners feel like members of that vocational community. Coxhead (2013: 117) assumes the point of view of Read (2007), who stated that ESP vocabulary research was not sufficiently systematic and, following Nation (2008), highlights the fact that very few statistical studies have been carried out on technical vocabulary. Earlier, it was believed that specialist vocabulary constituted approximately 5 percent of technical texts (Coxhead 1998 and Nation 2001, in Coxhead 2013: 118). However, Chung and Nation's study demonstrated that this number amounts to as much as 33 percent. In another study, Chen and Ge (2007, in Ferguson 2013: 254) discovered interesting correlations involving two lists of words: items from Coxhead's (2000) Academic Word List (AWL) and words frequently used in medical research articles (MRA): as little as 51.2 percent of AWL words appear in medical research articles (MRA); low-frequency MRA words have high frequency in the AWL. Based on this discovery, Wang et al.

(2008) produced a list of academic medical words. Their list was created using an analogous set of criteria as Coxhead's AWL. The result was a Medical Academic Word List (MAWL). Though not free of limitations, this list included 623 word families, which constituted only 54.9 percent of the AWL. This points to vast differences between the AWL and the MAWL.

Coxhead (2013: 117) offers a solution to establishing the scope of ESP vocabulary. This might be done through: consulting disciplinary experts, using technical dictionaries or categorization. Consulting disciplinary experts has several drawbacks, as different experts might have different opinions on word lists. On the other hand, technical dictionaries sometimes fail to resolve whether a given word is technical or not (Chung – Nation 2004: 254–255, in Coxhead 2013: 117). However, this method also heavily relies on the decisions made when constructing the dictionary. Coxhead reports that Chung and Nation's research showed that the dictionary approach accounted for 80% accuracy in determining the status of a word. Yet another technique is categorization. A given set of vocabulary items is categorized according some sort of a scale. We had an example of this in Salager's study (Basic English, Fundamental Medical English, Specialized Medical English). Following Salager, the main components of Fundamental Medical English are as follows:

- the word-compounding process, e.g. basement membrane thickening, blood vessel narrowing, iron-induced anaemia;
- the affixation process, e.g. limit – limitation – unlimited;
- the doublet phenomenon, e.g. kidney-failure vs. renal failure, heart failure vs. cardiac failure.

Creating compound nominal phrases is a process widely observed in many types of ESP. This allows for effective communication, especially that the English word order allows for stacking a number of adjectives in front of the key noun. Salager claims that in medical English we do not strive for synonyms but we would rather "resort to derivates" to avoid "inaccuracy". This tendency is not so clearly visible with ESP practitioners, who would rather treat the flexible use of synonyms as a sign of language competence, though synonym use is not something popular in within the IMRD writing format. The IMRD format itself has been investigated by many researchers, e.g. Antić et al. (2013: 424–428), Thompson (1999) or Paltridge (2002), among others (see the discussion in Flowerdew 2013: 349–350).

As Coxhead (2013: 118) claims, the saturation of text for specific purposes differs depending on the field of study. The ratio of general words to specialized vocabulary is 1 to 3 in anatomy and 1 to 5 in applied linguistics. Thus, we may attempt to determine the scope of ESP vocabulary on the basis of corpus linguistics. For example, in 1992 Atkinson (see Ferguson 2013: 28) investigated linguistic and rhetorical changes in medical journal articles discourse in the Edinburgh Medical Journal. The scope of changes embraced publications dating from 1735 to 1985. Also, numerous word lists in ESP have been developed on the basis of corpora (Coxhead 2013: 118–123), for example by Chen and Ge (2007) from a medical corpus of research articles with 190,425 words (Coxhead 2013: 121) or Wang et al. (2008 in Coxhead 2013: 122–123).

However, corpus-based studies mostly determine lemmas (single words) in frequency counts, while what is more interesting are lexical bundles, which are gaining popularity in ESP research as part of a wider research endeavour that looks into the nature of formulaic sequences or phrases (Coxhead 2013: 125–127). These would embrace, for example, a study by Pinna (2007) on multiword strings in dentistry or Grabowski's (2015) recent publication on phraseology in English pharmaceutical discourse.

It is important to stress that the corpus approach differs greatly from the categorization approach, with one approach examining the relationship between the function of the lexical items in the corpus and the other examining the closeness of the relationship between the words and the subject area.

Coxhead (2013: 123), following Hyland (2007) who investigated how words behave depending on the context, claims that medical learners need to develop specialized vocabulary early, and that the early specialization disciplinary-based approach is more appropriate than learning the general core first, and only then specialised vocabulary. Still, difficult decisions need to be made about vocabulary choice.

Apart from scientific names, there are many eponyms in medical English (Taylor 2005: 55–56) e.g. *Bright's disease, tetralogy of Fallot, Graves' disease, Raynaud's syndrome, Hodgkin's disease, Hippocratic facies* or *Paget's disease.* However, due to the high number of readers from various cultural and linguistic backgrounds, the tendency in medical writing is to use scientific terms. This might be explained by the globalisation of English. A scientific name is more understandable to the non-Anglophone audience, e.g. *von Recklinghausen's disease = neurofibromatosis, Caffey's disease = infantile cortical hyperostosis, relapsing febrile nodular nonsuppurative panniculitis = Weber-Christian disease.* Eponyms (Džuganová 2013: 63–65) named after the discoverers of a particular medical condition or the patients suffering from it are also very popular, e.g. *Parkinson's, Alzheimer's, Bartholin's gland, Fallopian tube, Addison's disease, Christmas disease, Hageman factor, Hartnup disease* or *Mortimer's disease.* The World Health Organisation recommends using multi-word terms rather than eponyms; however, they are very popular, to the extent that some medical conditions are named in contrast with them, e.g. non-Hodgkin's lymphoma. They can also be culture specific (Džuganová 2013: 65), e.g. *sideropenic dysphagia* is known under many names, such as *Plummer-Vinson syndrome* (US/Australia), *Paterson-Kelly's syndrome* (UK) or *Walderstrom-Kjellberg syndrome* (Scandinavia). One interesting form of eponyms used in English for Medical Purposes are toponyms (Džuganová 2013: 66), e.g. *Bornholm disease, Lyme disease, Ebola hemorrhagic fever or Stockholm syndrome* – all named after geographical locations. Mythonyms, e.g. *Achilles tendon, Oedipus complex, gigantism*, are becoming less popular (Džuganová 2013: 67).

There are many mistranslated medical terms and terms (Górnicz 2013: 140–142), e.g. *chronic* translated as *chroniczny* and not *przewlekły*, *epilepsy* translated as *epilepsja* and not as *padaczka*, to *take a history* translated as *przeprowadzić wywiad* instead of *zebrać wywiad*, *negative* translated as *negatywny* instead of *ujemny*. Also, *anaemia* is often translated as *anemia* instead of *niedokrwistość*. Górnicz (2013: 142–143) highlights the fact that there is no clear rule about transferring or reproducing English patterns, and that the prevalence of a given term should be studied on a case-by-case basis.

### 2.2.3 Core Grammatical Features of EMP

The relevance of grammatical accuracy for the needs of the globalized world of the lingua franca is a highly debated issue. The importance of grammatical accuracy in English for medical or biomedical purposes is also a bit of a conundrum. Due to the large amount of nominalizations used in EMP and high degree of text compression, it is often the case that readers of scientific papers are able to "extract" meaning from a text without paying much attention to grammatical cues. This tendency is especially visible in non-Anglophone users of English. Antić et al. (2013: 424–428) identified the following problem areas among non-native medical science communicators: subject verb agreement in the case of Latin-derived nouns and numerals, the choice of gerund vs. the infinitive, overuse of passive voice, the use of modal verbs for hedging, overuse of abstract nouns derived from verbs.

Rogers (2007: 39) makes a comment that it is often the case that scientific communicators play down the importance of "grammatical detail" for two reasons. Firstly, the effort put into attending to form is disproportionate/incommensurable to the appreciation from the readers. Secondly, most of the readers are non-native speakers of English. Learners of English often seem to function in the "lexical mode", in line with the Primacy of Lexis hypothesis. They seem to "enter" the analytical mode only when necessary.

#### 2.2.3.1 *Passivization and Personalization*

There are a number of studies on the use of particular language forms in the language of medical or biomedical writing – see the discussion in Basturkmen – Elder (2004: 675) or Ferguson (2013: 252) referring to research by Salager-Meyer (1994) on hedges, Carter-Thomas – Rowley-Jolivet (2008) on if-conditionals in conference presentations or Ferguson (2001) on if-conditionals in doctor-patient language. In his analysis of Health Communication Research, Ferguson (2013: 245) refers to earlier studies by Mintz (1992) and Anspach (1988) to enumerate some features of contemporary biomedical discourse: depersonalization, the use of agentless passives or existential 'there' constructions and the use of technology as agent.

Depersonalization is clearly demonstrated in the following examples: "The patient is a 21 year old Gravida III… black female 32 week gestation, by her dates. She states that…" (Anspach 1988: 363, in Ferguson 2013: 245) or "A 29-year-old woman, gravida 4, para 2, abortus 1 was seen on January 1, 19…, at 34 weeks of pregnancy" (Ciecierska, et al. 2004: 342). Whereas the tendency to treat technology as agent can be seen in: "Follow-up CT scan showed…" (Anspach 1988, in Ferguson 2013: 245).

The use of the passive voice in scientific writing has been a controversial issue for many years. Without doubt, the tradition of using the passive voice in scientific reporting is firmly engraved in scientists' brains. Many scientific communicators believe that it is inappropriate, even impolite, to use personal pronouns such as "I" or "we" (Rogers 2007: 68) and that passive sentences "are clearer" (Swales 1971, in Rogers 2007: 68) and "do not mention people", which might be confusing. Obviously, there are situations in which the passive voice does sound better (Taylor 2005: 41–42), e.g. "the patient was injected with the test drug" versus "we injected the test drug into the patient" or "the patient was transported to the hospital by ambulance" as this takes attention off the agent. These are legitimate instances of using passive constructions. However, the tendency to overuse the passive voice often stems from an unwillingness to use first-person pronouns (Rogers 2007, Taylor 2005: 41) because this means either assuming responsibility for the results of a study or because it is "erroneously regarded as impolite" (Taylor 2005: 41). Rogers (2007: 68) discusses the beliefs of scientific communicators concerning the use of the passive voice and concludes by saying that the tendency is "firmly engraved" to the extent that the use of personal pronouns is perceived as at best "inappropriate," and at worst "impolite".

Rogers postulates that, for the sake of clarity, the active voice should be used more often, and claims that most modern grammarians, linguists, and editors agree that the exclusive use of the passive voice is redundant (Rogers 2007: 68). According to Taylor, scientific writing is irrevocably moving toward an increase in the percentage of active voice used in medical writing, with active forms being more and more commonly used even in the most prestigious medical journals (Taylor 2005: 41–42), e.g.: "We followed up children once a day for diarrhoea and a month for anthropometry..." (*The Lancet* 2004(363): 112–118), "We enrolled 518 patients with polycythemia vera, ..." (*New England Journal of Medicine* 2004(350): 114–124), whereas in Polish medical writing it is still common to write: "...patients with ... were enrolled in the study". What is also highlighted by Li and Ge (2009, in Ferguson 2013: 249) is the tendency to use the first person plural pronoun "we," as there are more and more co-authored publications. The use of first person plural pronouns is consistent with the postulates for clarity.

### *2.2.3.2 Conditional Clauses*

The previously mentioned studies by Carter-Thomas and Rowley-Jolivet, as well as Ferguson's studies, demonstrate that if-conditionals do not constitute a substantial part of the linguistic means in EMP. Conditionals are used occasionally, with a higher incidence of subordinate if-clauses used to present the course of events. It comes as no surprise that "factual" conditionals are more popular in the Methods section and "hypothetical" conditionals in the Discussion section of IMRD papers, and non-conditional if-clauses are used in conference presentations "discourse management", e.g. "If you take a look at the median palliative index..." (Ferguson 2013: 253, after Carter-Thomas and Rowley-Jolivet 2008: 199). The main conclusion made by Ferguson is that learners should be made aware of both the forms and functions of a given structure. Ferguson also discovered that "polite directives" were more frequently used in doctor-patient consultations than in medical journal articles or medical journal editorials (Basturkmen – Elder 2004: 675).

### *2.2.3.3 Hedging*

Csongor and Rébék-Nagy (2013) investigated hedging in popular scientific articles on medicine, as a characteristic feature for EMP writing to show tentativeness and politeness. The authors were interested whether the amount of hedging was the same in medical research articles and in popularizations of medical research articles. The ratio of hedges in medical research articles varied from 1% to 2.2%. As far as popularizations are concerned, the authors obtained mixed results. They claim that numerical hedges, auxiliaries, epistemic verbs and adverbs were found in the corpus, although generally, due to the fact that popularizations are less tentative and use a more definite tone, hedges are rarely used. It is also often the case that the choice of reporting verbs, i.e. factive predicators for doctors (e.g. note, observe, record) and non-factive predicators for patients (e.g. claim, report, deny) highlights the objective-subjective perspective of doctor's accounts and of patient's accounts, the latter being perceived as subjective. Antić et al. (2013: 427) highlight the role of hedging is in medical discourse as "(…) the accreditation of knowledge depends on the consensus of the research community. Where evidence must be evaluated, and there is a need to comment on its reliability, hedging helps to avoid potentially hostile responses, and it may facilitate acceptance of research claims."

#### *2.2.3.4 The Use of Tenses*

As far as the use of tenses is concerned, medical interviews encompass both the use of present tenses – for present complaints, and past tenses – for past medical history and patient's history (Antić 2010: 160). The situation is different in medical articles, though as for many researchers the choice of tenses has to do with 'scientific ethics' (see Taylor 2005: 53, Rogers 2007: 41). What is acknowledged as "established knowledge" in the field, i.e. a) the general nature of the problem and b) background work on a given topic that has already been published in a primary journal (Taylor 2005: 203), should be communicated with the use of the present simple tense. This is no different from the notion of a "general truth" or "a law of nature" as we know it in General English, e.g. *HIV infection is highly prevalent in African countries.* (Rogers 2007: 41) or *In their groundbreaking work, Smith and Jones report a 33% survival rate in the test population* (Taylor 2005: 53).

What is acknowledged as "new findings" or "unpublished" data, i.e. the results of a study in question, should be communicated using the past simple tense, e.g. *We found that one third of the rats survived, one third died, and the third rat got away* (Taylor 2005: 53) or *Inhibition of the enzyme resulted in much higher plasma levels of the parent drug* (Rogers 2007: 41). Therefore, when researchers quote their own findings after they have been published, they can refer to them in the present tense as that information has already entered the "pool" of field-specific knowledge, e.g. *Inhibition of the enzyme results in much higher plasma levels of the parent drug* (Rogers 2007: 41).

As far as data description is concerned, perfect tenses are used in moderation (Rogers 2007: 42) as there is rarely an appropriate context to refer to, either "a moment in time before the reporting time point" or "a state of progression or a situation that is still existing", which would result in using past perfect or present perfect, respectively.

However, as Rogers (2007: 42–43) points out, the situation is not that simple in the Discussion section of the IMRD stylesheet, which allows for stating personal opinions (present tense, e.g. "We feel these findings indicate…"), further actions (future tense, e.g. "Further studies to examine the mechanism will be done").

*Table 2: Appropriate tense use in IMRD sections (after Rogers 2007: 43)*

| Context or section | APPROPRIATE TENSE |
|---|---|
| Established knowledge, previous results | Present tense |
| Methods, materials used, and results | Past tense |
| Description of tables and figures | Present tense<br>*Table 5 shows …; Figure 2 illustrates …* |
| Attribution | Past tense<br>*Jones et al. reported that …; Davies found …* |

*Table 3: Appropriate tense use (after Rogers 2007: 43)*

| Section | PREDOMINANT TENSE |
|---|---|
| Abstract / Summary | Past |
| Introduction | Mostly present tense (established facts, previously published data) |
| Materials / Methods | Past |
| Results | Past |
| Discussion / Conclusions | Mixture of past and present, sometimes future tense |

### *2.2.3.5 Sentence Complexity*

Even though clarity is crucial for effective writing, it is often the case that medical authors whose mother tongue is a language other than English have problems with information packaging within a sentence (Antić et al. 2013: 424, Rogers 2007: 1). Many authors are convinced that information load adds value to their papers (Rogers 2007: 10); however, as Taylor (2005: 42) highlights, medical sentences are often "jumbled and tortuous" due to the fact that medical communicators aim at putting as much information as possible into one sentence, to the extent that it becomes "barely intelligible".

What is more, medical sentences often seem to lack "action words". According to Taylor, the ratio of action words to words per sentence being 1:20 makes the sentence *weak* (Taylor 2005: 43–44) and proper "sentence density" prevents the sentence from becoming incomprehensible, e.g. *In addition to reduction in depressive symptoms, the intervention group compared with the usual care group at 12 months had lower mean (SE) scores for pain intensity (5.63 [0.16] vs. 6.15 [0.16]; between-group difference, _0.53; 95% confidence interval (CI), _0.92 to _0.14; P _ .009), interference with daily activities due to arthritis (4.40 [0.18] vs. 4.99 [0.17]; between-group difference, _0.59; 95% CI, _1.00 to _0.19; P _ .004), and interference with daily activities due to pain (2.92 [0.07] vs. 3.17 [0.07]; between group difference, _0.26; 95% CI, _0.41 to _0.10; P _ .002).*

Medical communicators often disregard the importance of verbs in a sentence, which often results in the lack of an action verb in a sentence. Taylor concludes by saying that many problems can be dealt with by a copyeditor, nevertheless, copyeditors, more often than not, do not happen to be experts in the field and have a hard time figuring out what the author meant to say (Taylor 2005: 62). To teachers of foreign languages, it comes as no surprise that Taylor (2005: 9) recommends reading good medical literature, e.g. the *British Medical Journal*, for the sake of style, as brevity and clarity should distinguish well-written papers (Antić et al. 2013: 424). Also, as far as the house styles of various medical journals are concerned, the choice of words in American journals does seem to be slightly different than that in European journals, e.g. *before* is used more often in British English and *prior to* in American English and articles need to be structured accordingly.

Both Taylor (2005: 54) and Rogers (2007: 73) disapprove of verbosity as far as the use of modifiers in EMP is concerned. Taylor claims that this is a tendency carried over from clinical note taking, where collecting detailed patient history is of crucial importance to the right diagnosis (e.g. wet and clammy, alert and responsive). Nevertheless, these do not need to be used in scientific publications, e.g. very frequently used similes (*cold as ice*, *pale as a sheet*) or expressions (*coffee-ground vomitus* or *cotton-wool exudates*) are indicative of certain disorders, but in formal writing can be replaced by more technical terms.

Sitkowski (2008: 26) provides interesting information on the issue of the technolect. He highlights the fact that the author and the recipients of a text need to use the same code, which is highly plausible in the context of medicine. What's more, English is a language that allows a high degree of text compression. Not only because many abbreviations used in laboratory tests are from English, but also because it is possible to put many descriptive words before the key noun, or create compound nouns. Górnicz (1997) distinguishes techniques used to decrease the number of words in a text, e.g. logical compression; syntagmatic or syntactic compression or terminological compression. Górnicz (2013:

142–142) gives an example of terminological compression: *A Smith Grade 3 patient* [patient with symptoms of the 3rd grade on Smith's scale] – *pacjent z objawami stopnia 3 w skali Smitha*.

One of the more interesting ideas for dealing with sentence complexity in professional discourse is postulated by the Plain Language Movement (see the discussion in, for example, Rogers 2007). The plain language movement is an attempt to demonstrate the benefits of writing clearly and concisely, in a reader-focused style. Founded in 1993, The Plain Language Association International, is an organisation whose aim is to:

> "Increase public awareness of plain language as a means of making communications from government, business, industry, the professions (including the medical, legal, information management, education and communications professions), and community organizations accessible internally and to a broad, public audience."
>
> (http://www.plainlanguagenetwork.org/networkindex.html)

Murray (1997: 351) discusses some very interesting psycholinguistic research on the impact of the clarity of instructions on the actions of jury members in the United States, resulting in drafting a specific pattern of jury instructions for civil court trials. Murray points to the possible sources of miscomprehension: the use of particular lexical items, the use of particular sentence structure, or the organisation of the text itself. The results of the study demonstrated a "significant improvement" in the level of comprehension "when traditional pattern instructions are rewritten based upon psycholinguistic principles of *simple English*" (Murray 1997: 348).

Appreciation for being able to pass on a message as effectively as possible dates back to ancient times, with Aristotle or Cicero already raising the issue. Effectiveness, does not imply simplicity or voiding language of all possible "ornaments", but rather the ability to skilfully intersperse them for better effect. In the first half of the 20th century, there was much research conducted on the principles of readability, as well as inquiries into the way the human mind processes and organises information. In 1975, Kincaid et al. came up with an algorithm that allowed to "predict the level of education required to read a selected text". The algorithm is known as the Flesch-Kincaid readability test, which takes into account word length as well as sentence length. More readability indexes accounting for subtleties were drawn up in subsequent years. Fascinating though the concept of readability is, this area of discourse studies will not be pursued in detail in this work. However, I find it interesting to mention that laws have been passed to facilitate the use of plain language, e.g. as of 2010, when The Plain Writing Act

(H.R. 946; Pub.L. 111–274) was signed by Barack Obama, federal executive agencies in the Unites States are obliged to put all documents into plain language.

Though the main interest of the Plain Language Movement seems to lie in legal English, there are many contributions to medical writing. Traces of it can be seen in the way medicine leaflets are composed. The European Medicines Agency provides guidelines for pharmacovigilance. I find the standardization of medicine leaflets and the focus being put on their comprehensibility to a lay reader a commendable manifestation of this tendency in medical writing, as well as the fact that more difficult medical terms have to be explained in brackets. Needless to say, miscomprehension of a piece of medical information might lead to a life-threatening situation.

Cook (2003: 66–67) brings up some issues connected with communicating new scientific research. Firstly, there is "the need to communicate (…) specialized knowledge to the outside world," i.e. a lay audience. According to Cook, this is done by means of two opposing tendencies: obfuscation and false clarity. Obfuscation is defined as "the failure to speak as plainly and straightforwardly as possible" (Cook 2003: 67). Cook claims that complexity might be an attempt to discourage anyone from investigating the matter. On the other side of the spectrum there is the "conversationalization" of professional discourse, which is not a good solution either as it might lead to oversimplification and imprecision.

#### *2.2.3.6 The Use of Prepositions*

Appropriate use of prepositions seems to pose a great deal of difficulty to many non-native health communicators. This is not only about the choice of prepositions, but also about the number of prepositions per sentence. As far as preposition choice is concerned, each EMP practitioner is probably able to come up with an extensive list of student errors in this area. Ribes et al. (2010) list some of the most typical errors regarding the use of prepositions:

* *The patient was operated with local anaesthesia.* (under local anaesthesia)
* *The cyst was 6 cm wide on the operative field.* (in the operative field)
* *Medial and collateral ligaments are well defined on the coronal plane.* (in the coronal plane)

As far as the number of prepositions per sentence is concerned, Rogers (2007: 71) discourages writers from using too many prepositions and recommends the ratio of prepositions to be 1:4 (4 words per preposition). Hence the sentence *The data from the participants of younger age in this study were compared with those of subjects of older age by an analysis of variance* (preposition ratio 8:25) is not as good as *The data from the younger and older study participants were compared by an analysis of variance* (preposition ratio 3:16, with *analysis of variance* as a fixed expression). As we can see, analysis of variance is one of many fixed expressions used in medical writing. Another area ridden with difficult fixed constructions are case reports, with phrases like: *on examination*, *the patients presented with*, *the patient complained of* (and not about) etc.

## 2.3 Doctor's English, Patient's English

Word choice decisions in healthcare communication often regard the convoluted issue of doctor or patient empowerment. When discussing or putting down symptoms, writing letters of referral to colleagues or delivering a diagnosis, doctors make genre-informed decisions. Quoting Mischler (1984), Ferguson talks about the problem of choosing the right register. It is a matter of choice between *the Voice of Lifeworld* and *the Voice of Medicine*. This argument is closely linked to the distinction between Anglo-Saxon and Latinate medical terms (Salager 1983) as well as colloquial words. Case reports, hospital discharge letters or conference presentations are only a few examples of situations in which doctors almost *retranslate* the patient's narrative into medical jargon. Following Hunter's (1991, in Ferguson 2013: 244) terminology, we can talk of the *incommensurability* of medical jargon and patient language. Nevertheless, due to the type of work they usually perform, healthcare providers should be versatile in both genre types: Doctor's English and Patient's English (Ribes et al. 2010: 3).

Non-native users of English for healthcare often find this area of communicative competence tremendously difficult, as this not only concerns commonly known "lay" names of popular diseases e.g. *mad cow disease* for *Bovine spongiform encephalopathy*, *avian flu* for the *H5N1virus* or *swine flu* for the *H1N1virus*, but most often about colloquial, or even slang names for body parts or symptoms.

Another problematic area is that EMP abounds in abbreviations and acronyms that are context and culture specific. Ribes et al. (2010: 177–179) provide an interesting classification of acronyms that, while it should be taken with a pinch of salt, nicely illustrates the phenomenon non-native healthcare professionals encounter in English-speaking work environments. These are: straightforward abbreviations, extra-nice abbreviations, expanded-term abbreviations, energy-saving abbreviations, multiple-meaning abbreviations and mind-blowing abbreviations, of which one of the most interesting examples is CABG (pronounced "cabbage") for coronary artery bypass grafting or CHOP (pronounced "chop") for a regimen of cyclophosphamide, hydroxydaunomycin, oncovin, and prednisone, used in cancer chemotherapy.

Loiacono (2013: 209) raises the important issue of doctor awareness of genres and conventions in medical communication, and concludes by saying that awareness-raising is what we should be developing in students. She also claims that most available materials are devoted to doctor-patient communication, whereas a lot of communication is happening among doctors and members of other healthcare professions, e.g. nurses, lab technicians or paramedics and that area should also be investigated.

## 2.4 Standardization of Medical Writing

There are many reasons why medical practitioners might want to commit themselves to writing. It might be to share ideas, express an opinion, generate discussion, assert "ownership" of a topic, enhance one's personal reputation, earn income or attain promotion, to mention just a few (Taylor 2005: 3). Whatever the motivation, the aim of medical writing is presenting facts and recording data. This is done mostly in the form of expository writing (Rogers 2007: 1; Taylor 2005: 105).

More and more courses are appearing, focusing on developing the skills necessary for facilitating doctor-patient communication. However, according to Ferguson (2013: 254) what is most needed globally at this stage of ESP development are courses in English for medical research. Good scientific writing is not only a matter of correctness; it is often just as much a question of good style and careful adherence to stylistic conventions used in a particular field of science (Rogers 2007: 67).

Scientific writing has undergone changes. Much has been done over the course of years to standardize scientific writing (Rogers 2007: 8; Loiacono 2013: 204). The European Medicines Agency guidelines, the IMRD stylesheet, the *British Medical Journal's* or *The Lancet's* guidelines or templates used by pharmacovigilance companies are an attempt to ensure clarity across different scientific domains, as clear communication on scientifically researched facts is not such an easy task. Many standards or tendencies, such as the use of the active or passive voice, were abandoned or modified over the course of years (Rogers 2007: 4). Generally speaking, following Rogers (2007: 1–2), good scientific writing is: understandable, transparent, clear, credible, efficient, simple and "devoid of unnecessary decorative words". Features such as clarity, simplicity, transparency or consistency are highly desirable if scientific communication is to be successful. This is in line with a radical view on English as a lingua franca, where "(…) for the purpose of international communication native speakers may need to adjust their language to a new norm" (Cook 2003: 9).

According to Rogers (2007: 4) clarity can be achieved by following some general guidelines. Some of them are consistent with the IMRD stylesheet and some of them are of a more general nature. IMRD does help to achieve a necessary degree of conformity. The aim has to be stated in an "obvious and unambiguous" way with consistent use of proper terminology throughout the paper. This is clearly stated in the IMRAD layout. The wording should be "grammatically correct, concise, accurate, and precise". The paper should have a logical structure and flow. Statements need to be anchored in recognized literature and congruent with the current state of medical knowledge and healthcare standards. Data presentation is also an important issue, as most conclusions are drawn from statistical analyses.

As, probably, with most academic fields, the abundance of publications makes it difficult to separate "the wheat from the chaff". To a discerning eye, this might be easy. However, to many non-native health professionals who might lack the proper linguistic judgment, the ability to pass a message on in such a way that the reader can "follow a train of thought" (Rogers 2007: 3) is what they wish to achieve. Grammar issues lag behind, unless they cause communication breakdown. Grammar issues come into play when the researcher's "face" is concerned. Who would like to have their paper dismissed on grounds of bad grammar? A poorly written paper may "jeopardize the credibility of the results. By extrapolation, it is our credibility as scientists that is at stake" (Rogers 2007: 7). Rogers claims that the judgment of the quality of a scientific paper lies with the readers (2007: 3). However, to my mind, it lies with a group of properly trained editors and providers of courses in academic writing. Proofreading a highly specialised medical publication requires both linguistic skills and a degree of understanding what one is reading. The editor must be versed both in language and medicine.

The baseline characteristics of a well-written paper incorporate correct grammar and spelling, as well as appropriate terminology. Style may refer either to the personal style of an author, or the house style of a given journal. As far as house style is concerned, most biomedical journals or publication houses follow the "Uniform Requirements for Manuscripts Submitted to Biomedical Journals: Writing and Editing for Biomedical Publication", first created by the Vancouver group. Stating opinions in biomedical publications also undergoes certain rules, e.g. when it comes to the use of tenses or hedges etc.

More and more journals require abstracts to be structured in a particular way, as only abstracts are available online free of charge (Ferguson 2013: 250).

Research analyzing the intricacies of medical abstracts is a popular trend nowadays (Ferguson 2013: 245). As Rogers puts it (Rogers 2007: 10), guidelines for authors, or stylesheets like IMRD have made it easier for the author to conform to certain standards, nevertheless the conviction that "quantity comes before quality" still seems to hold true. One might probably risk a statement that this approach is typical in other fields of science as well.

The situation is slightly different with case reports, another popular text type in medical writing. According to Ferguson (2013: 247–248) case reports have two characteristic features. They are a) essentially a narrative of a single case and b) recording the course of a patient's disease from diagnosis, through treatment to outcome. Developments in the field of medicine have led to a shift in the case report paradigm over the centuries. Ferguson gives an example of a study by Taavitsaianen and Pahta (2000) based on the analysis of case reports available in the *British Medical Journal* and *The Lancet* from 1850 to 1995. The following features were characteristic of 19^th^ century medical reports (Ferguson 2013: 248): a high degree of authorial involvement, some features of an oral mode of expression and abundant expressions of stance and effect, e.g. *I will now mention a case in which jaundice prevailed to a greater or lesser degree for eighteen months, with ultimate cure... He had some head-affection and was accordingly very strictly dieted: and to this restricted diet I impute his attack...* (Ferguson 2013: 248, after Taavitsainen and Pahta 2000: 64). This is far from what case reports look like nowadays. The development of clinical investigative methods and digitalization of work seem to have resulted in a change affecting case report discourse. Ferguson (2013: 248, after Taavitsainen and Pahta 2006) presents key features of 20^th^ century case reports: greater impersonality, achieved via increased use of passives and inanimate subjects, more frequent complex noun phrases, greater use of 3^rd^ person narrative, more uniform and conventionalized case report structure.

Case reports do not constitute as big a part of medical publications as they used to. Conference presentations regarding case reports only describe unusual cases. Nevertheless, writing case reports is an important skill to learn, as they require many formulaic expressions that cannot be substituted.

## 2.5 EMP Language Ability

As it is generally expected of health professionals to have "an effective command of English for medical purposes" (Charpy – Carnet 2014: 2–3), proper certification in medical English remains an open question. What is important in defining the notion of "ESP language ability" is the context and "desire for precision", with context being dependent on (after Hymes 1974) an interlay of factors such as the situation, participants, ends (purposes), act sequence (organization, content), key (tone), instrumentalities (language, medium), norms of interaction and genre.

Although the principles of assessment in ESP need not differ from the principles generally taken into account in language assessment, i.e. test purpose, test taker characteristics, target language use situation, test reliability or test validity (Douglas 2013: 367–68), ESP assessment must not evaluate subject specific knowledge but the ability to manipulate language functions appropriately (Davies 2001: 143 in Douglas 2013: 370).

> "(…) over the years, practitioners have gradually come to the realization that language knowledge and background knowledge are very difficult to distinguish in practice and that, although specific purpose testers are not in the business of assessing professional, vocational, or academic competence in specific purpose fields (Davies 2001), such competence is inextricably linked to language performance in those fields."
>
> (Douglas 2013: 369)

Domain-specific knowledge should be an important component of ESP assessment, not just for the sake of the face validity of a test, as Davies claims, but because domain-specific contextualisation of a task is what makes this type of assessment valid.

There exist internationally recognised profession-based language certification exams in business English (BULATS – Business Language Testing Service) or legalese (ILEC – International Legal English Certificate) or finance (ICFE – International Certificate in Financial English). There also exist many standardised language proficiency certification tests, but there is no uniform world-wide system of language certification for Medical Purposes. For example, in the United States, to obtain a license for practising medicine, foreigners need to take the United States Medical Licensing Examination (USMLE), in Australia the Occupational English Test (OET) is required, in Hungary a Proficiency Examination of English for Medical Purposes (PROFEX) is needed and in the United Kingdom they need to have a valid International English Language Testing System (IELTS) certificate (the academic version of the test, with a score of at least 7.0 in each testing area and an overall score of 7.5) as well as take a Professional and Linguistic Assessments Board (PLAB) test.

### 2.5.1 sTANDEM Certification

Assessing the language abilities of migrant healthcare professionals has become a real need in the European Union (see the discussion in Charpy – Carnet 2014: 3). This situation calls for standardised European testing. Thus, in 2011 there emerged an initiative called The European sTANDEM Project for Certification in Medical English. The aim of this EU funded project "is to standardise the requirements concerning skills in Languages for Specific Purposes (LSP) in medical settings all over Europe" (Charpy – Carnet 2014: 2). It is not to measure medical knowledge content, but the language skills of healthcare professionals whose native language is not English.

On a more technical note, Jacoby and McNamara tried to establish performance criteria for English for Medical Purposes claiming that the popular Occupational English Test (OET) did not cover on-the-job communication because "(…) using the traditional four linguistic skills to delineate special-purpose performance is inadequate to capture real-world communicative cultures and activities and that special-purpose performance is by definition task-related, context-related, specific, and local" (Jacoby and McNamara 1999: 234, in Douglas 2013: 371).

More and more researchers have started investigating the issue of ESP test design. Bakić-Mirić (2012: 31–33) highlights the importance of custom designed diagnostic tests in ESP courses and stresses the importance of qualitative feedback over quantitative assessment. She clearly supports the importance of formative assessment and carefully tailored diagnostic tests. In her paper, Anita Hegedűs discusses the intricacies and interrater reliability in the translation component of the C1 level PROFEX exam in English for Medical Purposes (Hegedűs 2013) and surprisingly finds holistic scoring to be more reliable than holistic and discrete point scoring combined.

Charpy and Carnet highlight the fact that generalist CEFR descriptors are not accurate for the assessment needed in LSP, and content "is a pre-requisite for successfully eliciting LSP performance" (Charpy – Carnet 2014: 4) in a profession-based examination. Medical certification needs to be distinguished from general certificates, as a high degree of test specialization adds to test accuracy and reliability. Also, it is crucial for test tasks to be authentic (Charpy – Carnet 2014, after Douglas 2000: 6).

The sTANDEM test was developed in such a way so as to assess the five language skills within a communicative CEFR-based, task-based, action-oriented paradigm and at the same time account for test validity and reliability in a professional context (Charpy – Carnet 2014: 6–7). For that purpose, the CEFR descriptors were re-written and tailored to provide more utilitarian tasks. Some of the changes are presented in *Table 4.*

The sTANDEM test developers encountered a number of problems when listing target key words or phrases, as well as the range of acceptable answers, often due to what was considered a transgression and what was still considered acceptable by the healthcare professionals community (Charpy – Carnet 2014: 7–8). Also, there were also problems with encompassing varieties of English (see *Table 5*).

*Table 4: CEFR descriptors tailored to the sTANDEM project*

| | Listening comprehension | Reading (two texts – longer and shorter) | Writing (Tasks 1 and 2) | | Speaking (Tasks 1–3) |
|---|---|---|---|---|---|
| B1 | patient information,<br>health reports, undergraduate lectures | textbook extracts, product descriptions, information leaflets | job applications, invitations, congress applications;<br>analysing a diagram and giving factual information | introductory conversation about the job and/or research field of the candidate | a simulation of a doctor-patient conversation focusing on history-taking |
| B2 | interviews with healthcare professionals, patients, and caregivers, medical news reports,<br>case reports, graduate lectures | official letters on professional topics, specialised case reports,<br>referral letters, extended abstracts, application letters | cover letters,<br>referral letters,<br>complaint letters;<br>giving factual information and interpreting messages | | a talk on the basis of a diagram, table or graph |
| C1 | postgraduate medical lectures and talks,<br>research reports, conference presentations,<br>case studies | research articles, letters to the editor, ethical approvals editorials, informed consent statements, reading peer reviewers' comments | letters to the editor, case reports, answering reviewers' comments<br>giving factual information, interpreting and arguing | | a simulated interview between a healthcare professional and a patient arguing and/or explaining<br>a short presentation on a professional issue |

There were also problems with medical terms, or their "common English" counterparts fitting the CEFR scale (Charpy – Carnet 2014: 8), e.g. terms *barking cough* or *excruciating* seemed too difficult for the B1 CEFR level, but are crucial for proper history taking. Another frequently encountered issue was redesigning test items in such a way so that the test takers would not be able to answer the question or fill in a gap on the basis of their knowledge of medicine (Charpy – Carnet 2014: 9–11).

*Table 5: Sample terminological issues*

| | GB | US |
|---|---|---|
| lekarz | doctors | physicians |
| | physicians<br>(surgeons vs. physicians) | |
| wcześniak | premature baby | preemie |

Similarly, in the United States Medical Licensing Examination (USMLE) the candidate needs to provide the correct answer to clinical cases on the basis of a short description of patient history, signs, symptoms or laboratory findings etc. It is often the case that inability to understand the sentences prevents them from choosing the right diagnosis. To my mind, such test design provides better language screening than demanding IELTS or TOEIC from non-Anglophone healthcare professionals (see the discussion in Eggly et al. 1999 or Read – Wette 2009). Basturkmen and Elder (2004: 672) are of the same opinion, i.e. that a shift towards "contextualised performance-based measures" of testing ESP has to take place. Also, many valuable insights into the assessment of language skills in international medical graduates (IMGs) is provided in a recent publication edited by Hoekje and Tipton (2011) with a focus on the issue of acculturation as well as the linguistic aspect of success in interactional achievement.

To conclude, test design of ESP tests should differ from test design of generalist English tests. Also it would be reasonable for English for Medical Purposes tests to belong to the so-called 4$^{th}$ generation tests, i.e. tests "which foster a learning mode that is close to real life and require language skills integrated into easily-identifiable cognitive and discursive learning processes likely to be developed before the administration of the test" (Tardieu 2013: 246, in Charpy – Carnet 2014: 11). It is the combination of language activity and content knowledge that leads to a successful completion of a task that is authentically representative of the target situation (Douglas 2000, in Johns – Price-Machado 2001: 48).

## 2.6 Concluding Remarks

Specialist competence allows the learner to function in a domain-specific context, usually a workplace. The goal of learning and teaching English for Medical Purposes is to enable successful communication on all three levels of specialist competence: linguistic, discursive and intercultural (see Grucza 2013a). Although the role of terminology in ESP is unquestionable, research shows, that the aim of ESP teaching is to find a balance regarding the choice of lexical units, elements of grammar, as well as language functions based on the specific needs of the learner. This is a choice, at best, made by means of corpus-informed decisions.

# Chapter Three: Motivation, Learner Autonomy and the Role of the Teacher in Learning and Teaching English for Medical Purposes

## 3.1 Motivational Dimensions

It is important to look at the dynamics of language learning from the perspective of the intricate relationship between factors such as motivation, learner autonomy or the role of the teacher in the ultimate success or failure in learning English for Medical Purposes.

The discussion of motivation and its influence on learning achievements in the educational context has been wide an extensive, e.g. Berliner – Calfee (1996), Boekaerts (2001), Brophy (1987), Burden (1995), Canfield – Wells (1994), Covington (1998), Cook – Singleton (2014), Damon – Eisenberg (1998), Dörnyei (1994, 2001, 2005), Dörnyei – Csizér (1998), Dörnyei – Schmidt (2001), Dörnyei et al. (2014), Galloway et al. (1998), Good – Brophy (1994), Kikuchi (2015), McCombs – Pope (1994), McDonough (1986), Oxford–Shearin (1994), Pintrich (2003), Pintrich – Schunk (2002), Scheidecker – Freeman (1999), Schunk et al. (2008), Williams – Burden (1997), Wlodkowski (1986), Wolters (2004) and Zybert (2006, 2012), among others.

Sections on motivation can be found in the majority of ELT teacher training coursebooks e.g. Brown (2000), Cranmer (1996), Chambers (1999), Larson (2009), Leaver et al. (2005), Leibling and Prior (2005), Lightbown and Spada (1993), Komorowska (2005) or Ur (2009), among others.

Motivation is the force that drives the human effort in its quest to achieve the desired objectives and determines their outcome (Zybert 2012: 103). The questions of "why" (the choice of a particular action), "how hard" (the effort expended on it) and "how long" (the persistence with it) someone will pursue a given goal or an activity have been central to the concept of motivational theory and research for several decades now (Dörnyei 2001: 6, Brown 2000: 160). Diachronically, Dörnyei (2005: 66) divides research into L2 motivation into: the social psychological period (1959–1990), the cognitive-situated period (during the 1990s) and the process-oriented period.

Initially, motivation was investigated by Biggs (1976, 1978, 1979) and Gardner and Lambert (Gardner 1979, 1985; Gardner – Lambert 1959, 1972) and it changed throughout the 20th century, depending on developments in the field of psychology (see the discussion in Brown 2000: 160, Dörnyei 2001: 7–11). Freud attributed motivation to instincts and drives, behaviourists such as Pavlov or Skinner stressed the significance of the stimulus-response reaction, and the anticipation of reward or punishment, humanistic psychologists regarded the self-actualising tendency as a crucial motivational factor, whereas within the cognitive approach it was the individual's attitudes and beliefs that propelled actions. Constructivists, on the other hand, stressed not only individual choices but also the social context for motivation.

Following Ausubel (1968: 368–379, in Brown 2000: 160), human actions are driven by a number of needs, i.e. the need for exploration, the need for manipulation (understood as operating), the need for activity, the need for stimulation, the need for knowledge and the need for ego enhancement. Following Maslow (1970), motivation is strongly related to the hierarchy of human needs, i.e. needs to satisfy physiological needs, the individual's safety needs, feelings of belonging, self-esteem issues and, on top of that, the need for self-actualization. Dörnyei (2001: 9) speaks of "the multitude of potential determinants of human behavior" influencing "a relatively small number of key variables that would explain a significant proportion of the variance in people's action." It should perhaps be noted at this point that educational psychologists are not eager to offer one-size-fit-all recommendations.

Based on a longitudinal follow-up of a group of college students, McClelland (1965, in Coon – Mitterer 2007: 406) identified a "need for achievement variable" (*nAch*) that accounts for making life choices. People with low *nAch* are more willing to choose "sure things" or "impossible goals" so that they would not have to assume responsibility for possible failure. People with high *nAch* are more willing to achieve excellence in their occupations, as well as "attribute success to their own ability, and failure to insufficient effort." The approach to motivation based on the belief that it is innate for humans to have the need to meet goals and objectives, and that we can distinguish high- and low-achievers, is known under the name of achievement theory (see McClelland 1965, Atkinson 1957).

The theory that accounts for the causes people attribute to achievement (success) or lack of it (failure) was developed by Weiner (1974) as well as Kelley and Michela (1980) under the name of attribution theory. Attributions such as "ability", "effort", "task difficulty" and "luck" (see *Table 6*) are assigned within a matrix of categories, including stable – unstable (stable theory), internal – external (locus of control) as well as controllable – uncontrollable (controllability).

Deci and Ryan's (1986) self-determination theory of motivation and personality, which laid the foundations for research into types of motivation, explicates human behaviour as dependent on the necessity to meet three basic, innate psychological needs, that of competence (need to achieve mastery), relatedness (need to interact with other members of the community) and autonomy (need to be in charge of one's life).

*Table 6: Weiner's attribution matrix (after Zybert 2012: 112)*

| cause | internal | external |
|---|---|---|
| **stable** | *ability* | *task difficulty* |
| **unstable** | *effort* | *luck* |

The 1990s saw a growth in interest in bridging the concept of motivation in educational psychology with the field of foreign and second language learning (see the discussion in Crookes – Schmidt 1991: 469, Dörnyei 2001, Williams – Burden 1997, among others). There are many perspectives on motivation in the foreign language learning context. Schumann's (1986) acculturation theory, Gardner and Lambert's (1972) motivation theory, Clément's (1986) theory of linguistic self-confidence, self-determination theory, attribution theory, Dörnyei and Kormos' (2004) task motivation theory, Dörnyei and Ottó's (1998) process-oriented representation of motivation or neurobiological theories of motivation all aim at accounting for learner behaviour (see the discussion in Cook – Singleton 2014 or Dörnyei 2005, among others). Research into attributional patterns ("causal attributions") relating the learner's past learning experiences to future efforts was another important concept in the search for phenomena accounting for success or failure in foreign language learning (Dörnyei 2005: 79–80). Yet, even though there is no doubt that motivation is one of the key issues in successful foreign language learning, practitioners in the field of ELT might get the impression that the overall picture is "fragmented" and this lack of synthesis is not conducive to effective classroom practice (Dörnyei 2001: 10–12).

> "The real problem with motivation, of course, is that everyone is looking for a single and simple answer. Teachers search for that one pedagogy that, when exercised, will make all students want to do their homework, come in for after-school help, and score well on their tests and report cards. Unfortunately, and realistically, motivating students yesterday, today, and tomorrow will never be a singular or simplistic process."
>
> (Dörnyei 2001: 13; after Scheidecker – Freeman 1999: 117)

Motivation was no longer discussed irrespective of the foreign language classroom context but viewed through its prism. Dörnyei distinguishes three levels (1994, 2001) of foreign language learning motivation: the language level (referring to concepts of culture and community as well as integrativeness and instrumentality), the learner level (referring to Clément's notion of self-confidence) and the learning situation level (referring to classroom setting). The learning situation level comprises course-specific motivational components (i.e. syllabus, the teaching materials, the teaching method and the learning tasks), teacher-specific motivational components (i.e. impact of the teacher's personality, behaviour and teaching style/practice) and group-specific motivational components (i.e. characteristics of the learner group).

On terminological grounds, it should also be noted that Brown (2000: 163) makes an important distinction between orientation and motivation, as motivation can be high or low within the scope of a given orientation. With this in mind, nevertheless, the term "motivation" will be used throughout this chapter to denote "the impetus to create and sustain intentions and goal-seeking acts" (Cook – Singleton 2014: 90).

## 3.2 Types of Motivation

### 3.2.1 Intrinsic and Extrinsic Motivation

The concept of intrinsic and extrinsic motivation, with intrinsic motivation defined as "the desire to engage in behaviours for no reason other than sheer enjoyment, challenge, pleasure, or interest" and extrinsic motivation as relying on "external rewards and encouragement" (MacCallum 2009) was developed within Gardner and Lambert's (1972) socio-educational model.

The term intrinsic motivation was used to denote activities "for which there is no apparent reward except the activity itself" (Deci 1975: 23, in Brown 2000: 164), or actions performed "without any obvious external rewards" (Coon – Mitterer 2007: 407). Whereas, in contrast, in the case of extrinsic motivation, activities are performed "in anticipation of a reward from outside and beyond the self" as well as "to avoid punishment" (Brown 2000: 164) and they "stem from external factors" (Coon – Mitterer 2007: 407). The intrinsic – extrinsic motivation dichotomy is sometimes brought up regarding the "play" and "work" distinction. Performing some actions is considered enjoyable and a reward in itself, and performing others a chore that has to be rewarded somehow (Coon – Mitterer 2007: 407). In a similar vein, Williams and Burden's framework (1997, in Dörnyei 2001: 19) offers a division into internal and external motivation.

A body of research points to intrinsic motivation as more effective (see the discussion in Brown 2000: 164). This innate pursuit for "self-actualization" (see the discussion in Coon – Mitterer 2007) is in line with Maslow's (1970) hierarchy of needs, Piaget's (1952, 1972) idea of intrinsic simulation, Hunt's (1965) optimal incongruity as a powerful motivating factor, or Krashen's (1985) "i+1" zone of proximal development. It has also been demonstrated that excessive extrinsic incentives seem to decrease intrinsic motivation (Lepper et al. 1996, Green – Lepper 1974, Tang – Hall 1995).

In the case of institutionalized learning contexts, the students are "forced towards and placed in an educational milieu, which forms a *forced ecosystem*," which due to "historically and culturally justified popular consent, has been designed to promote learning and diffusion of knowledge" (Puppel 2012: 8). However, from the point of view of language learning methodology, it is important to find the balance between a reasonable amount of external/extrinsic incentives and the skilful development of internal/intrinsic motivational orientation, e.g. in the case of students who are obliged to take English for Medical Purposes classes. As it is often the case that extrinsically motivated learners choose "the fastest, most direct route to a goal, not the most creative" (Sternberg – Lubart 1995, in Coon – Mitterer 2007: 408). Puppel (2012: 9) rightly points out that what ought to be accomplished in a "positively-oriented" foreign language learning pedagogy is a "positively-loaded *thriving* framework" and not just a "merely *surviving* framework". Mobile assisted foreign language learning might add to this framework and enrich classroom practice for the educational process to thrive.

### 3.2.2 Integrative and Instrumental Orientation

Gardner's (1972, in Dörnyei 2001: 16) motivation theory is based on a dichotomy of integrative and instrumental motivation (*Figure 4*).

Integrative motivation is defined in literature as a "socially or culturally oriented" (Brown 2000: 163) "positive disposition toward the L2 group" (Dörnyei 2001: 16) and its "way of life" (Cook – Singleton 2014: 95) which leads to developing a sense of community with the target language speakers.

Instrumental motivation is defined in the literature as an "academic or career-related" (Brown 2000: 163) situation in which "language learning is primarily associated with the potential pragmatic gains of L2 proficiency" (Dörnyei 2001: 16) and a "desire to obtain something practical from studying a second language" (Cook – Singleton 2014: 96).

*Figure 4: Motivation dichotomy (after Brown 2000, Dörnyei 2001)*

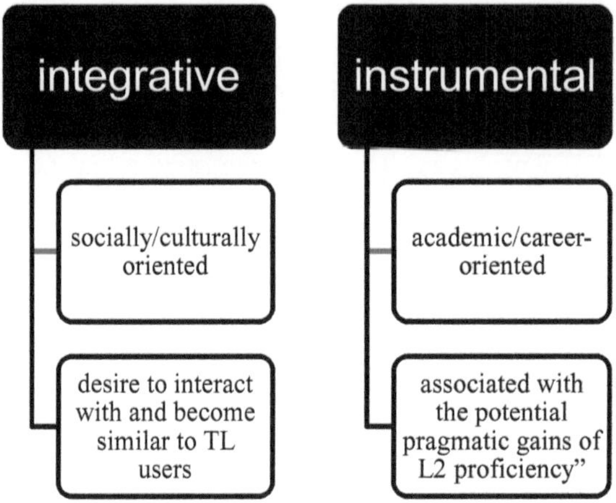


Whereas initially it was believed that integrative motivation leads to better learning results (Gardner – Lambert 1972, Spolsky 1969), a number of researchers challenged that assumption (Lukmani 1972, Au 1988, Gardner – MacIntyre 1991). Now it is generally acknowledged that there is no single best type of motivation, and foreign language learning rarely takes places in purely integrative or purely instrumental contexts (Brown 2000: 163). The integrative and the instrumental orientation are not mutually exclusive (Cook – Singleton 2014: 96). More often than not, learning contexts usually encompass a combination of motivational incentives, illustrated in a well-known motivational matrix presented in *Table 7* (Bailey 1986, in Brown 2000: 166).

*Table 7: Motivational matrix (Bailey 1986, in Brown 2000: 166)*

| | **Intrinsic** | **Extrinsic** |
|---|---|---|
| *Integrative* | L2 learner wishes to integrate with the L2 culture (e.g., for immigration or marriage) | Someone else wishes the L2 learner to know the L2 for integrative reasons (e.g., Japanese parents send kids to Japanese-language school) |
| *Instrumental* | L2 learner wishes to achieve goals utilizing L2 (e.g., for a career) | External power wants L2 learner to learn L2 (e.g., corporation sends Japanese businessman to U.S. for language training) |

More recent motivational matrixes are offered by Ushioda (2001) and Noels (2003). The former encompasses eight motivational dimensions, whereas the latter draws on research by Ushioda to present three dimensions (*Table 8*).

*Table 8: Motivational dimensions (after Ushioda 2001 and Noels 2003)*

| Ushioda (2001) | Noels (2003) |
|---|---|
| Actual Learning Process<br>• Language-Related Enjoyment/Liking,<br>• Positive Learning History<br>• Personal Satisfaction | Intrinsic Reasons Inherent in the Language Learning Process |
| External Pressures/Incentives | Extrinsic Reasons for Language Learning |
| Integrative dimension<br>• Personal Goals,<br>• Desired Levels of L2 Competence<br>• Academic Interest<br>• Feelings about French-speaking Countries or People | Integrative Reasons |

The challenges of a globalized world led Gardner to redefine his motivation theory. In his revised model, Gardner distinguishes three components within the socio-educational model: integrativeness, attitudes and motivation (Gardner 2006, in Cook – Singleton 2014: 97). It is a combination of these factors, i.e. degree of identification with the target language community, attitudes towards the target culture and the amount of effort put into the learning process, that differentiate between successful and unsuccessful foreign language learners.

At this point perhaps a word or two should be said about the notion of integrativeness, with a focus put on it in the ESP context. The intensity of integrativeness can range from "a moderate desire to socialize with" to a "need to identify" with target language speakers (see Brown 2000: 164). In this book, integrativeness will be defined following McClelland (2000: 109, in Dörnyei 2005: 95) as "integration with the global community rather than assimilation with native speakers".

*Figure 5: Gardner's conceptualisation of the integrative motive (after Dörnyei 2001: 17, Dörnyei 2005: 69)*

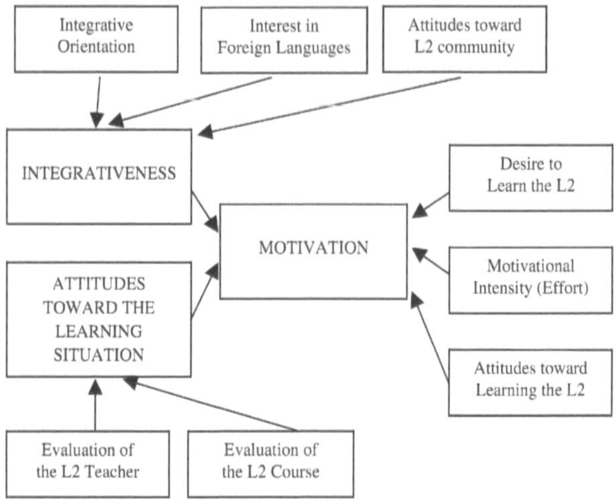


### 3.2.3 Other Theories of Motivation

Motivation causes actions to be initiated, sustained, directed, and terminated (Petri 2003). Dörnyei (2001) points to the importance to account for "changes of motivation over time" in the learning process as "motivation cannot be viewed as a stable attribute of learning that remains constant for several months or years." It is thus important to add a temporal axis to the model. Motivational flux is a widely observed phenomenon (see Dörnyei 2001: 29). It is clear that motivation levels fluctuate depending on the circumstance the learners find themselves in (Cook – Singleton 2014: 98). It is the role of the teacher to sustain appropriate levels of motivation.

Williams and Burden (1997: 121, in Dörnyei 2005: 83) distinguish the following motivational stages: 1) reasons for doing something, 2) deciding to do something and 3) sustaining the effort, or persisting. Motivation must be "actively nurtured," as initial motivation tends to fade away if not sustained. In order to sustain learner involvement Dörnyei (2001: 71–72) suggests, e.g. "breaking the monotony of learning", "making the tasks more interesting" or "increasing the involvement of the students". But first and foremost, a framework to categorize motivational teaching practice, i.e. creating the basic motivational conditions, generating initial motivation, maintaining and protecting motivation as well as encouraging positive retrospective self-evaluation (Dörnyei 2001: 28–30, Dörnyei 2005: 86).

Furthermore, an important element of "linguistic self-confidence" was added to the motivational theory by Clément et al. (1994, in Dörnyei 2005: 73–74) as foreign language learning success or failure may be to a great extent determined by self-perceptions of L2 competence, as for example in the case of self-conscious learners.

Various models were created to account for reasons behind, intensity fluctuation in, and trajectories of motivation in the foreign language learning context. Yet the above mentioned models were generated focused on traditional and not mobile learning contexts. The following section will discuss motivation in the context of mobile assisted language learning.

## 3.3 Motivation in Mobile Learning

Research into motivational dynamics regarding the influence of technology on the learning process has a relatively long history, e.g. Malone (1981). Motivation in broadly understood technology-enhanced learning contexts is discussed by numerous researchers, e.g. Breen – Lindsay (2002), Conole et al. (2008), Demb et al. (2004), Hall – Elliott (2003), Herrington (2009), Herrington et al. (2009), Keller (2008), Kuo (2005), Lane – Yamashiro (2008), Laurillard (2002, 2007), MacCallum (2009), MacCallum – Jeffery (2010), Martin (2006), McMillan–Honey (1993), Newhouse (2001), Ng – Howard (2016), Oberg – Daniels (2013), Oloruntoba (2006), Roberts (2005), Roblyer – Doering (2010), Seifert – O'Keefe (2001), among others.

It is a common preconception that the very introduction of technology (and m-learning in particular) in teaching practice will generate intrinsic motivation among learners (e.g. Laurillard 2007: 156; Roblyer – Doering 2010, in Martin 2013: 52). It is generally assumed that learning tools operating in the mobile environment increase student motivation and engagement in the learning process (Attewell – Webster 2004, in Marcos et al. 2010: 1069). Researchers often highlight a relationship between positive attitudes towards the use of technology in educational contexts and intrinsically motivated goal orientedness among students – see the discussion in MacCallum (2009), Åkerlind – Trevitt (1999), Kennedy et al. (2008), Bouhnik – Marcus (2006) or Liaw (2008), among others. Many learners are attracted to mobile devices as they offer substantial control over learning goals, contexts, continuity etc. but, seemingly more important, also usually provide a considerable amount of fun, which plays an important role in "harnessing" technology for learning (Jones et al. 2006).

In general, students who are more tech savvy are also reported to be more independent learners, and the other way round, both leading to greater willingness to adopt new technologies in the learning process. Although recent studies suggest that it is no longer always the case that "students will be naturally motivated to use mobile devices for learning" (Martin et al. 2013: 52).

*Figure 6: The relationship between computer literacy and willingness to adopt new technologies for learning*

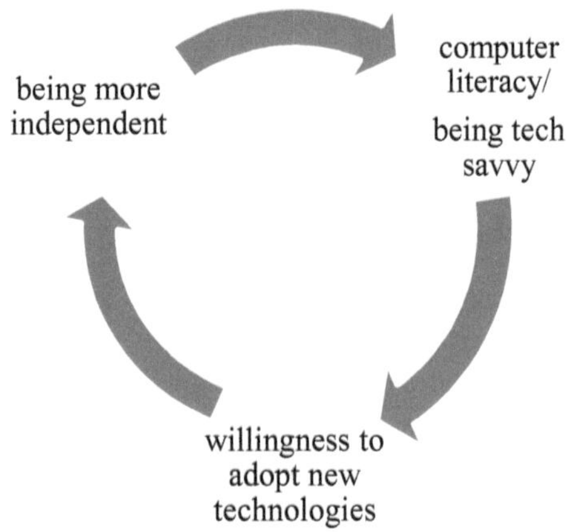


Sharples (2006) characterizes the young generation in Europe as owning at least one or more mobile computers and communicators, and often engaging in rich networking and online learning activities. A generation that often regards classroom-based learning as "a distraction from their rich informal activities" (Sharples 2006: 21) and a generation requiring m-learning to enable them to obtain relevant information "as they want it and when they want it" (Kukulska-Hulme – Shield 2008: 280), preferably in a "bite-size" approach with study material broken into smaller chunks distributed over time (Hoppe 2006: 32). No wonder then that among the factors relevant for mobile learning Jones et al. (2006: 16) list not only control (over goals), ownership, privacy, instant access, sharing or portability, but also communication, learning-in-context, continuity between contexts coupled with fun and identity ("coolness"). Dias (2002) argues that some learners may reject m-learning because they perceive it as an intrusion into their personal lives, rather than a help. All of which poses a challenge to mobile design, not only at the educational concept level but also at the level of the interplay between an educational idea and "down-to-earth" technical orchestration and technological constraints (Hoppe 2006: 33). Supporting m-learning in an effective way thus involves integrating the elements of bite-sized learning, individualization and studying at one's own pace.

*Figure 7: Factors affecting motivation in m-learning*

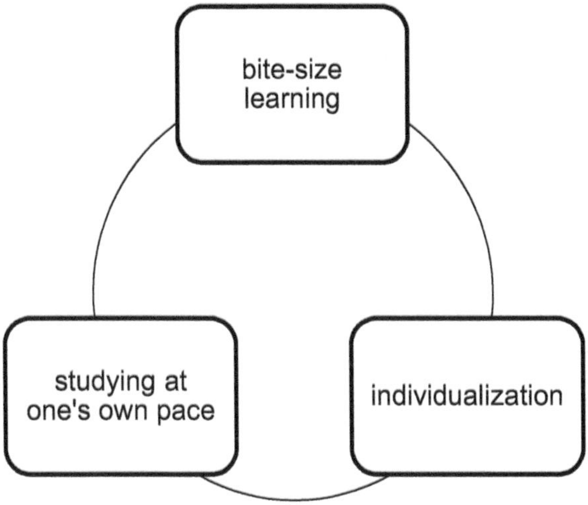


A sufficiently high level of motivation is required to accomplish long-term goals (Dörnyei 2005: 65). In the case of m-learning with the use of flashcard spaced repetition software, motivation needs to be actively nurtured on the level of software solutions. Following Dörnyei (2001: 75) "boring but systematic" teaching might suffice to achieve desired short-term effects, whereas it is not sufficient to "inspire a life-long commitment to the subject". Motivational strategies, i.e. techniques that encourage the individual's goal-related actions, and more precisely techniques "consciously exerted to achieve some systematic and enduring positive effect" (Dörnyei 2001: 28) need to be embedded within the program itself, as learning usually takes place in an informal context. State-of-the-art IT solutions facilitate not only providing learners with information, but also offer sophisticated ways to support the learning process.

It is often repeated that the novelty factor plays an important role in the perception of CALL or MALL activities. Compared to traditional pen-and-paper tasks, technology-enhanced tasks appear attractive to learners, leading to higher ask satisfaction rates, although for some learners technology-enhanced learning decreases "coping potential," as they are afraid they will not be able to cope with the task due to lack of computer literacy. Schumann's (2000) neurological theory of stimulus appraisal (see the discussion in Dörnyei 2005: 92–93), embracing the "emotional relevance" and "motivational significance" of mental processes, attributes the motivational surge to the following incentives: novelty, pleasantness, goal/need significance, coping potential as well as self and social image. Among ways of making tasks more interesting, Dörnyei (2001: 76–77) enumerates: challenge, interesting content, the novelty element, the intriguing element, the exotic element, the fantasy element, the personal element, competition, tangible outcome and humour.

The Memrise designers and developers aimed to incorporate the above mentioned factors into their software solutions. The "Leaderboard" solution adds to the gamification and competition among learners who can climb through a series of ranks (*Table 9*). It is also possible to "follow" other Memrise users and verify your achievements against theirs.

*Table 9: Memrise ranks (adapted from* http://www.memrise.com/thread/1291880/*)*

| **Memrise ranks: unofficial list** | |
|---|---|
| Member | 0 |
| Memdicant | 2,000 |
| Memorandum | 5,000 |
| Memtor | 10,000 |
| Mempee | 25,000 |
| Memsahib | 50,000 |
| Memonimee | 100,000 |
| Memblem | 200,000 |
| Memmoth | 250,000 |
| Memocrat | 500,000 |
| Membrain | 1,000,000 |
| Memonist | 2,000,000 |
| Membassador | 5,000,000 |
| Meminence | 10,000,000 |

Dörnyei (2001: 77–84) discusses personalizing learning tasks and setting personal learning goals, claiming that "goal-setting dramatically increases productivity" (see the discussion in Locke – Latham 1990, in Dörnyei 2001: 82) and "goal setting can have exceptional importance in stimulating L2 learning motivation" (Oxford – Shearin 1994: 19, in Dörnyei 2001: 82). As evidence, Dörnyei recalls a study by Bandura and Schunk (1981, in Dörnyei 2001: 83) on goal setting in a maths course where students with the most precisely specified goal had the best results. Goals set for students should be clear and specific, measurable, challenging and difficult but also realistic. They should also have a fixed completion date, be divided into short-term and long-term goals. Memrise offers a gradation of learning goals to accomplish daily, from the threshold level of 1,500 learning points to a score of 6,000 points, to the level of 20,000 points daily, which corresponds to 5, 15 and 45 minutes of daily learning, respectively. Tangible effects in the form of, for example, completing a daily goal three days in a row are rewarded with a special "badge" visible in the user's profile (a solution similar to, for example, badges awarded in Edmodo classes).

The fantasy element, the intriguing element and the humorous element seem to be embedded in the "mem" creation mode, with "mems" defined as "anything that helps you create a connection between a word and its meaning" (http://feed back.memrise.com/knowledgebase/articles/524873-what-is-a-mem) On technical grounds, "mems" can be composed of photos, images, GIFs, videos, vines (short-form looping video clips) but also sentences or quotations as "[t]he only end goal of a "mem" is to enrich your learning by helping you commit something to long term memory in an enjoyable, vivid way."

## 3.4 Learner Autonomy

Interest in learner autonomy, or the lack of it, influenced the field of linguistics throughout the 20th century, with behaviourist, cognitivist, constructivist and humanistic views on the nature of human behaviour. Language education was influenced by developments in psychology, e.g. research into individual differences in language learning or research on motivation. The concept of learner autonomy evolved with the developments in applied linguistics and the interests of researchers and teachers themselves (Zybert 2012: 159). Attempts were made to identify features of a good language learner (e.g. Rubin 1975, Rubin – Thompson 1982, Naiman et al. 1995). The 1960s saw the implementation of mnemonic strategies in the educational context. The learner was no longer perceived as a passive recipient but as "an active, self-determined individual who processes information in complex ways" (Dörnyei 2005: 188). Learner autonomy, defined as "(…) the capacity to take control over one's own learning" (Benson 2013: 2), was first introduced to language teaching with the rise in interest in lifelong learning, the birth of the Council of Europe's Modern Languages Project (1971) and the involvement of Yves Châlon and Henri Holec in the development of the Centre de Recherches et d'Applications en Languages, i.e. CRAPEL (Benson 2013: 9). Soon, there appeared the first self-access learning centres, providing learners with an abundance of learning materials. Self-access centres to a great extent fed on developments in educational technology, and quickly became computer-assisted (Benson 2013: 10–11). As a result, the 1980s and 1990s saw a rise in research into learner strategies (e.g. Learner Strategies for Leaner Autonomy by

Wenden (1991, in Benson 2013: 12). The idea slowly gave rise to the notions of learner-centeredness and the necessity to meet the needs of individual learners or, as in ESP, groups of learners of different professions. Nowadays, learner autonomy is a topic widely discussed in the literature and ELT coursebooks (e.g. Benson 2001, 2013; Dörnyei 2001; Lamb – Reinders 2005, 2008; Little 1993, 1995, 1997, 2007a, 2007b, 2008, 2009a, 2009b; Watkins 2005 and Zybert 2011, 2012, among others).

The concept of learner autonomy has both proponents and opponents. It is perceived as either "a distraction from the real business of teaching and learning languages" or "a precondition for effective learning" (Benson 2013: 1). In his publication, Benson discusses many aspects of the relevance of learner autonomy to the process of foreign language learning and teaching, as well as the current state of research in the field of learner autonomy. Most researchers would agree that "(…) autonomy refers to the learner's broad approach to the learning process, rather than to a particular mode of teaching or learning" and "(…) autonomy is in essence multidimensional and takes different forms in different contexts of learning" (Benson 2013: 1). Also, Benson (2013: 4) claims that, in a fast-developing world, we should rather talk of language learning autonomy as epitomizing broader personal autonomy, which would be congruent with some of the results obtained in the research project discussed in Chapter Five.

Moreover, the technological developments of recent decades brought "an increased interest in and need for the development of learner independence in all its forms" (Lamb – Reinders 2005), which in turn resulted in a number of challenges for foreign language teachers, researchers and educational institutions. Computer- or mobile- assisted language learning enables learning to take place "independently of the teacher" in terms of time and place. However, independently does not necessarily mean "without the control of the teacher" (Lamb – Reinders 2005). Greater learner mobility and flexibility results in greater demand for being able to make decisions concerning the "when," "where" and increasingly often "what" to study. Although, as Zybert (2012: 158) highlights, this does not mean that the teacher becomes redundant to the student. On the contrary, the teacher is indispensable in the process of developing learner autonomy, because autonomy is more about the cooperation between the teacher and the student than about self-education (Zybert 2012: 161).

Surprisingly, the above-mentioned control over learning goals, listed as an m-learning motivational factor (Jones et al. 2006: 16), is strongly connected with the idea of informal interest-led education. While appropriation and user centred design of mobile learning tools allow a considerable degree of freedom over the learning process, nevertheless, most learners feel the need to verify the learning process somehow. One of the attempts to effectively support that need was an application that, by means of student self-assessment, provided data to "exert some control over the expected result of the learning process" (Marcos et al. 2010).

Much is known about developing learner autonomy in institutionalized learning (*Table 10*). The question that arises is whether the theories of motivation usually applied in non-mobile contexts apply to mobile contexts as well (see the discussion in Jones et al. 2006). Or as Davies (2009: 267) puts it, do mobile applications encourage students to become self-regulated learners who know how to manage learning resources, learning time, motivation and strategies?

*Table 10: Activities that foster autonomy (Benson 2001, in Dörnyei 2001: 107)*

| | |
|---|---|
| Resource-based approaches | independent interaction with learning materials<br>individualised learning<br>peer teaching |
| Technology-based approaches | independent interaction with educational technologies |
| Learner-based approaches | direct production of behavioural and psychological changes in the learner, e.g. strategy training |
| Classroom-based approaches | changes in the relationship between learners and teachers in the classroom and learner control over the planning and evaluation of learning |
| Curriculum-based approaches | extend the idea of control over the planning and evaluation of learning to the curriculum as a whole |

Memrise facilitates the development of learner autonomy at the resource-based level (as defined by Benson 2001), allowing individualised learning and independent interaction with learning materials through personalized accounts, as well as peer teaching, thanks to the crowdsourcing "mem" mode and user created content. It also promotes the development of learner autonomy at the technology-based level by independent interaction with educational technologies through mobile and handheld devices. What is more, Memrise influences learner autonomy at the learner-based level by triggering and entrenching changes in learning habits. It encourages learners to take more and more control over the learning process and in this way shape their commitment to learning.

Loiacono (2013: 209) claims that medical students tend to demonstrate analytical skills in learning strategies and enjoy step-by-step logical learning. They enjoy sequencing, protocols and procedures. Based on that premise, it might be assumed that they might also derive a considerable amount of pleasure from "growing one's own garden of memory" – as advertised by Memrise.

## 3.5 The Role of the Teacher in EMP

What is characteristic of ESP is the nature of interaction that takes place between the ESP practitioner and his/her learners (Dudley-Evans – St John 1998). It resembles more of a teacher-learner partnership than the traditional provider-recipient classroom relationship.

Dudley-Evans and St John (1998: 13–17, in Paltridge – Starfield 2013: 19) enumerate five functions of an ESP practitioner: teacher, course-designer and materials provider, collaborator (often with a subject or vocational specialist), researcher and evaluator. Nevertheless, in the ESP classroom, in many cases, the learner is an expert in his/her field, whereas the teacher is often an expert in language and an enthusiast, interested in a given topic. The teacher rarely is an expert in the field or a guru who *lifts the veil of secrecy* about the content matter. This point is also raised by Belcher (2013: 545), who highlights the intricacy of the teacher-learner relationship in ESP.

Thus, one of the most vexing issues when examining the roles of ESP practitioners is the question of whether they ought to be experts in the field. According to some, only experts should teach a given variety of ESP. On the other side of the spectrum, we have graduates of English studies specialising in teaching methodology and familiar with the intricacies of the language system that may be unknown to non-linguists. It seems that not expert knowledge, but the readiness *to be flexible and to take risks* plays an important role in the success of the individual ESP teacher (see the discussion in Dudley-Evans – St John 1998: 14, Belcher 2009a: 2). This is approach is also supported by Ferguson, for whom even if the teacher does not teach specific terminology, they can be of great assistance as far as scaffolding the process is concerned. Non-field-expert ESP teachers can develop proper pronunciation or "(…) equip students with strategies for learning such vocabulary: for example through fostering students' skills in recognizing technical words, interpreting definitions, and relating word senses to core meaning" (Ferguson 2013: 254, after Chung – Nation 2003).

Belcher (2013: 544–546) highlights the fact that there is little research on teacher efficacy in ESP, and complains about very few preparatory courses being available for prospective ESP practitioners. As far as ESP courses are concerned, teachers often have a difficult task to fulfil, trying to introduce to their students the discourse of a community they are not necessarily a member of (Parkinson 2013: 156). That is why ESP practitioners who are also experts in a given field are of such value to the process. Unfortunately, in the case of medical English, practising doctors are rarely linguists as well, and are rarely interested in teaching ESP courses.

It is more often the case that doctors go abroad and polish their knowledge of English in target language contexts.

Mackiewicz (2004) claims that it is often the case that humanities-trained writing tutors do not provide appropriate advice to students of engineering, for example. On the other hand, Górnicz (2013: 131) argues convincingly that linguistic competence does not boil down to knowing vocabulary equivalents, but being versatile in genre conventions is of great importance as well. Górnicz (2013: 134) highlights that opinions about non-expert translators vary from "it is all in the dictionary" to "only a subject specialist can translate a text properly". Górnicz counters the latter opinion, saying that many legal documents are translated by court-appointed translators who do not need to be experts in the field of law and that the translator's work experience is of far greater importance. Therefore, projecting this discussion onto the ESP teaching field, ESP teachers do not need to be experts in the field and what counts more is familiarity with the subject matter, and knowing the concepts behind the terminology and not possessing a licence to practice the art of treatment (Górnicz 2013: 135–144). Nevertheless, it is clear that a close degree of cooperation between the ESP teacher and an expert in the discipline is desirable (Horn et al. 2008), as, for example, in the case of Labov and Hanau's (2011) project aimed at improving the pronunciation skills of non-native English-speaking pathologists.

English for Medical Purposes courses offer valuable insight into the teacher – medical expert interaction. As defined by Dakowska (2005: 152), the former creates the primary conditions for foreign language learning as well as facilitates and catalyzes the process of foreign language learning in the educational setting, whereas the latter provides an invaluable source of content knowledge.

English for Medical Purposes education at university level offers a limited amount of class time of 90 minutes of instruction per week. Thus, most learning activities crucial for successful foreign language learning take place without the presence of the teacher. Learners need to be less reliant on the teacher, who thereby becomes more of a teaching process manager, using all three functions of mobile technologies, i.e. administration, reference and interactive functions (Herrington 2009, after Patten et al. 2005) in the learning process.

## 3.6 Concluding Remarks

What this chapter has looked at is the role of motivation and learner autonomy, as well as the teacher in the process of foreign language learning. It seems that instrumental motivation may play an important part in achieving a threshold level of language proficiency, but integrative motivation is needed to develop language mastery. Motivational theories aim at explaining the driving force behind human actions. McClelland's research on the high and low achievement variable, and the motivational flux theory coupled with linguistic self-confidence theory might shed some light on the motivational conundrum regarding ultimate success or failure in foreign language learning. However, nowadays, learning takes place in so many contexts and spaces that the idealistic belief that "all students are motivated to learn under the right conditions, and that you can provide these conditions in your classroom" has become outdated (McCombs – Pope 1994:vii, in Dörnyei 2001: 25). Since so many learners are attracted to mobile devices (Jones et al. 2006), new solutions need to be developed to support language learners throughout the mobile assisted language learning process (Shepherd 2001). The ubiquity of smartphones, their portability and convergence make them an appropriate tool to do so (Herrington 2009: 135–136).

Noels (2001) demonstrated a direct correlation between teachers being perceived as controlling and a decrease in intrinsic motivation among their students. Also, it was shown that extrinsically/instrumentally motivated learners were less susceptible to the teacher's instructional style causing self-determination or enjoyment. Developing learner independence makes learners assume responsibility for the learning process, and learner involvement in the process is a key prerequisite for learning to take place in the first place. What is more, to promote long-term vocabulary retention, it is essential to promote efficient out-of-class language learning. The concept of learner autonomy is strongly rooted in a conviction that learning should be self-directed and self-motivated. According to Sha et al. (2012, in Martin et al. 2013) mobile learning, apart from enabling student-centred, personal and ubiquitous learning experiences, perhaps more importantly, "requires learners to be motivated and to self-regulate their learning". First year medical students fall into the category of Early Adult Transition as defined by Corder (2002: 3). As learners who have attended primary and secondary level schools, they have developed a number of skills and collected various learning experiences. It is a common belief that medical students are highly apt, internally motivated and conscientious learners, and as such should be willing to undertake actions to enhance their knowledge and competencies (see the discussion in MacCallum 2009). Motivation is crucial for any self-directed learning (Garrison 1997). Self-directed and independent learners are likely to engage and succeed in online learning contexts. Based on this premise, my research project aimed at evaluating whether they would be willing to adopt a new technology, and enjoy the challenge of learning English for Medical Purposes via flashcard spaced repetition software, and whether being motivated means being successful in learning English for Medical Purposes. More explicit control over the learning process on the part of the learner requires more flexibility on the part of the teacher, who assumes the role of a facilitator. Many researchers highlight teacher development as a key tenet for successful m-learning – see the discussion on teacher development in Ellis et al. (2010). Having examined the relationship between autonomy and motivation, it is reasonable to assume that "the freedom to choose and to have choices (...) is a prerequisite to motivation" (Dörnyei 2001: 103). For that reason, part of the research project was conducted in the voluntary mode. Also, MacCallum (2009) distinguishes four dimensions influencing the success of failure of m-learning: general ICT experience and attitudes, motivation, learner dependence as well as attitude to mobile learning. Following Seifert and O'Keefee (2001, in Martin et al. 2013: 52) it is of crucial importance for students to feel confident, have a sense of control over their learning and consider learning activities to be meaningful and relevant. The question arises whether Memrise satisfies these needs as a learning tool. In the discussion of motivation in the educational context, an interesting perspective opens up in connection not just to learner autonomy but also self-regulation as a broader concept (Dornyei 2005: 190), with self-regulation defined as "the degree to which individuals are active participants in their own learning" (Dornyei 2005: 191). In mobile assisted language learning the handheld device becomes a ubiquitous "personal learning hub" (Wong et al. 2010) offering a plethora of opportunities for those learners who are keen to engage in learning. To those who are keen, but perhaps demonstrate weaker self-regulatory capacity, or those who are not keen but required to learn, online educational tools offer a scaffolding, e.g. in the form of scheduled reminders or daily/weekly or monthly goals.

The ultimate goals of developing learner autonomy are to reduce learner dependence on the teacher. An important argument is made by Zybert (2012: 155) that although no one disputes the beneficial effect of formal education on the results obtained by learners, it is not clear to what extent teaching is actually effective, and how much depends on the student's commitment to the learning process itself. Therefore, it seems important to provide data on whether Memrise fosters degrees of motivation and engagement sufficient for learners to achieve to their potential. Informed by Breen and Lindsay's (2002) study, who demonstrated that across various discipline areas students may require different motivators, and that to some students the enjoyment associated with a learning experience might be more important than completing learning goals, in Chapter Five, I discuss the efficiency of the course content of Memrise-based learning of English for Medical Purposes.

# Chapter Four: Key Tenets of Mobile Assisted Language Learning

## 4.1 Introduction

This chapter offers an overview of the current state of mobile learning research and practice, with specific reference to Mobile Assisted Language Learning (MALL). It also delineates various dimensions of mobile learning and mobile applications as mediating tools in the learning process, with special focus on flashcard vocabulary tutors.

Technological advancement is taking place at an unprecedented rate (Attewell 2005, Herrington 2009, Mac Callum 2009) leading to improved access to mobile devices (Lefoe et al. 2009: 17). We can observe a rapid growth in smartphone use throughout the developing world, and numerous mobile learning projects across Europe (Walker 2006: 3). Mobile phones ranked first among devices used in mobile learning projects funded by the European Union (Pęcherzewska – Knot 2007, in Kukulska-Hulme – Shield 2008: 271–274). And they have been gradually gaining popularity and recognition in both small and large educational contexts, e.g. BBC Bitesize Mobile, MOBILearn European Project (Sharples 2006: 2).

The world we live in requires developing lifelong learning skills, which judging by the pace of life and the omnipresence of handheld devices, in turn requires designing learning in such a way so as to answer the needs and wants of learners, especially in a situation where technology allows producing a variety of digital content "on the spot" (Milrad 2006).

For many learners engagement and interaction through technology are an essential aspect of their lives (Lefoe et al. 2009: 25) and yet mobile technologies are not widely or routinely used in education (Herrington 2009: 28).

> "While this mobile/wireless computing revolution is having a major impact on the ways people communicate and interact, this transformation does not live up to the promises and expectations when it comes to schools and universities."
>
> (Milrad 2006: 28)

The availability of mobile devices does not translate into their use in learning contexts and still little theoretical foundation is available on how to use mobile devices for pedagogical purposes (Herrington et al. 2009: 1).

## 4.2 Definitions of Mobile Learning

Broadly speaking, mobile learning (m-learning) can be defined as "any form of learning that happens when mediated through a mobile device" (Herrington 2009: 1). Early definitions of mobile learning defined it by the tools used, whereas more recent definitions focus on the "anytime, anywhere" (Geddes 2004) aspect of m-learning, and its being "independent of location and space" (Quinn 2000, in Lefoe et al. 2009: 17) as well as the fact that it allows students to "(…) overcome restrictions of time and space, enabling learners to study whenever and wherever possible" (Chen – Chung 2008: 625).

Some researchers classify m-learning as an extension of e-learning, whereas others insist that it is an independent field with a focus placed not on its technological aspect but it being location- and situation-independent (see Nyiri 2002, McLean 2003 in Marcos et al. 2010). Mobile learning is defined as "taking place when the learner is not in a fixed, predetermined location" (Lefoe et al. 2009: 17) or when a learner "takes advantage of the learning opportunities offered by mobile technologies" (O'Malley et al. 2005: 6, in Lefoe et al. 2009: 17). Traxler highlights the importance of "any educational provision where the sole or dominant technologies are handheld or palmtop devices" (Traxler 2005). Following Trifanova et al. (2004: 3, in Kukulska-Hulme – Shield 2008: 273) it is important that the devices be "(…) small, autonomous and unobtrusive enough to accompany us in every moment". Lefoe et al. (2009: 18) offer yet another definition of m-learning as "[p]ersonal access to mobile technologies providing learners with opportunities to be flexible in the way they collect, store and share information to support their problem solving."

Kukulska-Hulme and Traxler (2007: 182) offer a distinction of m-learning types into: technology-driven mobile learning, miniature, but portable e-learning, connected classroom learning, and informal, personalized, situated mobile learning.

*Table 11: M-learning typology after Kukulska-Hulma and Traxler (2005: 182)*

| | |
|---|---|
| technology-driven mobile learning | specific technological innovation deployed in an academic setting to demonstrate technical feasibility and pedagogic possibility |
| miniature but portable e-learning | mobile, wireless and handheld technologies used to re-enact approaches and solutions already used in 'conventional' e-learning (...) merely using mobile technologies as flexible replacements for static desktop technologies |
| connected classroom learning | the same technologies are used in classroom settings to support collaborative learning |
| informal, personalized, situated mobile learning | the same technologies are enhanced with additional functionality, for example location-awareness |

Current perspectives on mobile learning (Winters 2006: 5–6) stress the importance of four aspects of m-learning: technocentricity, relationship to e-learning, augmentation of formal education, and learner centredness.

The technocentric approach, with m-learning defined as learning with the use of a mobile device, seems to be the most popular approach currently. M-learning is also often characterised in relation to e-learning, i.e. as a type of e-learning, with a high degree of learner mobility, or as opposed to traditional forms of classroom-based learning (*Figure 8*).

*Figure 8: Classification of educational spaces (after Kuzmicz – Skrzydlewski 2012: 82)*

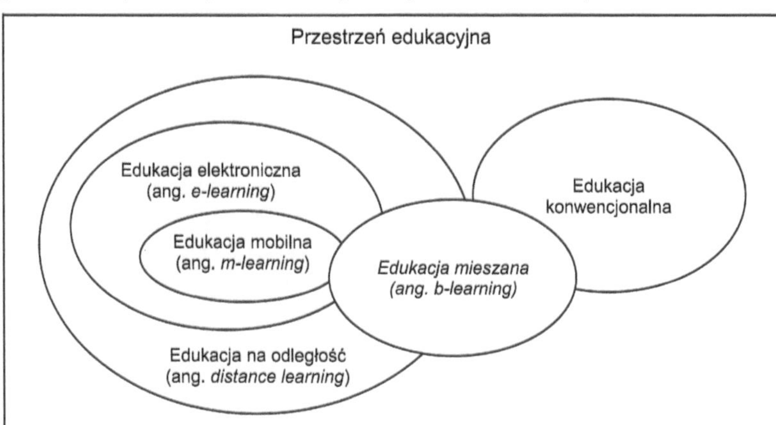

However, what seems to be the most promising approach to m-learning is its link to the concept of learner-centredness, as it is not the device, but the learner "on the move" that is a necessary condition in this educational equation. Walker (2006: 3) makes an important claim that there is more to mobile learning than simply using portable devices. The crux of the matter is learning across contexts.

> "Mobile learning is not something that people do; learning is what people do. With technology getting smaller, more personal, ubiquitous, and powerful, it better supports a mobile society."
>
> (Walker 2006: 3)

From a theoretical standpoint, m-learning applications "are underpinned by many theories of learning" (Winters 2006: 5). MALL can be approached either from a content-based or design-related perspective (see the discussion in Kukulska-Hulme – Shield 2008: 273) but it is rarely underpinned by a coherent theory of mobile learning. With some critical voices concerning m-learning definitions, e.g. Winters (2006: 5) postulating the need to redefine m-leaning as it is currently too vague a concept, the latest definitions emphasize the role of the learner, rather than the role of technology and highlight the instrumental role of the devices, as well as the need for MALL solutions to comply with second language pedagogy.

## 4.3 Review of Research on M-learning

In recent years, the concept of mobile assisted learning has gained prominence in the field of educational research. There is a growing body of literature concerning m-learning, as various forms of mobile learning and their implementation in the educational context have been explored by researchers and educational practitioners, e.g. Åkerlind – Trevitt (1999), Andrews (2003), Arrigo et al. (2013), Attewell (2005), Belanger (2005), Bouhnik – Marcus (2006), Caudill (2007), Chang et al. (2003), Chen – Chung (2008), Chinnery (2006), Collins (2005), Corbeil – Valdes-Corbeil (2007), Cortez – Roy (2012), Demouy – Kukulska-Hulme (2010), Demouy et al. (2010, 2013), Farrow et al. (2010), Gajek (2015), Gaved et al. (2013, 2014), Geser (2004), Jones et al. (2006), Kennedy et al. (2008), Kim et al. (2006), Kukulska-Hulme (2005, 2006, 2007, 2008a, 2008b, 2008c, 2009a, 2009b, 2010a, 2010b, 2010c, 2010d, 2010e, 2012a, 2012b, 2012c, 2013a, 2013b, 2013c, 2014), Kukulska-Hulme – de los Arcos (2011, 2015), Kukulska-Hulme – Bull (2008, 2009), Kukulska-Hulme – Jones (2011), Kukulska-Hulme – Petit (2007, 2008, 2009), Kukulska-Hulme – Sharples (2016), Kukulska-Hulme – Shield (2008), Kukulska-Hulme – Traxler (2005, 2007), Kukulska-Hulme – Wible (2008),

Kukulska-Hulme et al. (2007, 2009a, 2009b, 2010, 2011a, 2011b, 2015a, 2015b), Leung – Wei (2000), Liaw, (2008), Lu (2008), MacCallum (2009), McCombs – Liu (2006), McNicol (2005), Miller – Piller (2005), Milrad (2006), Naismith et al. (2004), Norbrook – Scot (2003), O'Malley et al. (2005), Pachler (2007), Paletta et al. (2013), Park (2006), Pearson et al. (2014), Perry (2003), Petit – Kukulska-Hulme (2007, 2008, 2011), Pecherzewska – Knot (2007), Pownell (2006), Proctor – Nurton (2003), Rogers et al. (2005), Scanlon et al. (2005, 2014), Scott et al. (2006), Seta et al. (2014), Sharples (2000, 2005), Sharples et al. (2002, 2007), Shield – Kukulska-Hulme (2008), Smith – Kukulska-Hulme (2012), Thornton – Houser (2002), Traxler (2005), Vavoula et al. (2009), Winters (2006) or Wood (2004), among others.

A recent overview of research projects dealing with m-learning can be found in, e.g. the *Handbook of research on M-learning methodologies for Language Acquisition* (de Cássia Veiga Marriott – Lupion Torres 2009) or on a list of 345 MALL projects dating from 1994 to 2012 compiled by Burston (2013) which might serve as a lynchpin for those interested in MALL implementations. It is expected that m-learning will add value to the educational process and enable more efficient instruction (Marcos et al. 2010: 1069). Below, I will present some research projects of interest with regard to the research project discussed in Chapter Five.

The beginnings of m-learning research date back to the pre-smartphone era, and concentrated on the use of text-messaging and mobile phone conversations in the learning process. Stanford University was one of the first research facilities investigating the use of mobile phones in the process of language learning (Brown 2001). The results obtained demonstrated, for example, that students in a Spanish study program preferred announcements obtained by SMS rather than e-mail or web-based. The study participants enjoyed learning vocabulary via text-messaging, as well as mobile-mediated quiz delivery. Stanford University also set up a project involving learners being coached by native speakers over the phone, as well as a project in which learners took automatic voice-controlled quizzes. Cooney and Keogh (2007, in Kukulska-Hulme – Shield 2008) describe a study in which mobile phones and iPods were used to listen to and record answers to questions that were later marked by teachers. Dias (2002a, 2002b, in Kukulska-Hulme – Shield 2008) describes the use of a web-board, and a mailing list accessible by mobile phone. Motiwalla (2007, in Marcos et al. 2010) conducted a study on the usefulness of WAP technology, such as RSS news alerts, in university education. City College in Southampton (Kukulska-Hulme – Shield 2008) ran a research project involving the use of "media boards" for problem-based tasks.

Technological developments over the last few years have opened the way to a plethora of research projects involving not only mobile technologies but smartphones in particular. Kiernan and Aizawa (2004) explored the use of mobile phones in task-based learning, providing data showing the statistically significant better performance of mobile phone learner users over computer users. Fallahkhair et al. (2007) developed a platform which embraced both mobile phone use and interactive television to provide immersive content available for learning "on the move". Herrington (2009) describes a research project in which digital narrative episodes were created with the use of a smartphone as a data collection tool. The goal of the project was to assess the technological and pedagogical affordances enabled by the use of a smartphone. Rau et al. (2008, in Marcos et al. 2010) discovered that the use of short text messages decreased the "experience of pressure" among secondary school students. Kennedy and Levy (2008) studied the acceptability of text messaging to support vocabulary learning, with special focus on the *push* mode of operation where learners received scheduled messages. Ruchter et al. (2008, in Marcos et al. 2010) pointed to the fact that m-learning may facilitate incidental learning. Scanlon et al. (2005) investigated the use of mobile technologies in informal contexts. Kukulska-Hulme and Shield (2008: 272) examined the extent to which mobile devices "can support listening and speaking activities in situations where learners may wish to collaborate". Chen (2010, in Marcos et al. 2010) investigated mobile peer- and self-assessment systems. Herrington and Herrington (2007) explored the use of mobile devices in higher education, with focus on pedagogy for mobile devices. Marcos et al. point out that there are only a few comparative studies regarding m-learning at different educational levels (Marcos at al. 2010: 1070).

The idea pervading in m-learning research is that of how to best capitalize on the fact that MALL enables users to personalize the learning experience within the institutional constraints of educational facilities.

## 4.4 The Nature of Mobile Learning

Among the wide range of technologies implemented for language teaching and learning (Garrett 2009: 719), mobile devices can have great educational value (see the discussion in Hoppe 2006). Phones were used to provide feedback as well as assistance to language learnersas early as in the 1980s. Nowadays, with technical limitations slowly being eradicated, mobile learning is a step towards the idea of a "wireless campus" (Kukulska-Hulme – Traxler 2005: 181) as well as self-directed life-long learning in informal learning contexts. This section is an attempt to delineate the unique dimension of mobile learning.

The notion of m-learning as opposed to traditional study environments is widely discussed in the literature (see the discussion in, e.g. Cobcroft et al. 2006, Corbeil et al. 2007, Gulek – Demitras 2005, Ingleton et al. 2000, Kim et al. 2006, Sha et al. 2012, among others) and is backed up by a number of studies on the implementation of mobile devices, such as e.g. mobile phones or laptops in educational contexts (e.g. Hall – Elliott 2003, Keller 2008, McCallum 2009, McMillan – Honey 1993, Newhouse 2001, Oloruntoba 2006).

Whereas the early generation of mobile assisted language learning offered activities that were meticulously designed by educators and engineers, nowadays, due to widespread access to mobile devices, mobile assisted language learning is more likely to be used to support social contact and promote collaborative learning (Kukulska-Hulme – Shield 2008: 271, Kukulska-Hulme et al. 2007, Petit – Kukulska-Hulme 2007). Thus, it seems that it is not a matter of preparing versions of existing activities that the relatively small screens of mobile phones would support, but rather of adopting different learning scenarios and approaches to shape the educational experience itself.

> "M-learning transcends the barriers between in-class and out-of-class experiences with opportunities for anywhere anytime learning and the potential for students to participate in educational activities beyond the limitations of traditional study environments."
>
> (Martin et al. 2013: 51)

Patten et al. (2006, in Herrington 2009: 28) distinguish a number of educational contexts in which mobile devices can be used, e.g.:

- Administration, e.g., calendars, exam reminders, grading software;
- Referential, e.g., dictionaries, e-books and office applications;
- Interactive, e.g., quizzes, response software;
- Microworld, e.g., simulations, games;
- Data collection, e.g., data logging, note taking, audio recording, eportfolios;
- Location aware, e.g., augmented environments, GPS navigation and tagging;
- Collaborative, e.g., pod/vodcasting, blogging, instant messaging.

And although conventional e-learning also functions in these educational contexts, what distinguishes mobile assisted language learning (MALL) from computer assisted language learning (CALL), is "use of personal, portable devices that enable new ways of learning, emphasizing continuity or spontaneity of access and interaction across different contexts" (Kukulska-Hulme 2008: 273). However, although we distinguish CALL from MALL, with the growth of functionality of devices, greater processing speed and storage, it is becoming easier and easier to move resources across devices, and thus the boundaries between these two categories are becoming blurred. With ongoing technological development, MALL has the potential to influence foreign language learning and teaching, especially once drawbacks such as small screen sizes, internet access or data transmission speed have been overcome. Nevertheless, even with its obvious limitations, for the time being, m-learning clearly offers a number of solutions inaccessible to conventional e-learning (Kukulska-Hulme –Traxler 2005: 181).

Numerous researchers are exploring the nature of the informal learning experience in the context of "a society on the move" with the decreasing impact of formal classroom-based learning. In "a society on the move" m-learning seems to be an extension of e-learning that is better suited to empower learners (Sharples 2006).

> "Any sort of learning that happens when the learner is not at a fixed, predetermined location, or learning that happens when the learner takes advantage of learning opportunities offered by mobile technologies"
>
> (O'Malley et al. 2003)

Mobile learning easily allows education to extend beyond the classroom context (Sharples 2006: 2). The use of handheld mobile devices can support learner engagement as well as offer greater choice in the activities learners can take part in (Kukulska-Hulme – Traxler 2005: 180). One of the more important aspects of m-learning is also its informal, *out-of-class use* (Fallahkhair et al. 2007, Trivfanova – Ronchetti 2003: 1796, in Kukulska-Hulme – Shield 2008: 278–279). Mobile based learning (MBL) is likely to take place in the informal learning context, e.g. in the learner's spare time or waiting time (Morita 2003: 1, in Kukulska-Hulme 2008: 278). It has also been suggested that, for this reason, m-learners have "highly fragmented" attention, and thus they should be offered short, "bite-sized" learning modules (30 seconds to 10 minutes).

Following Kukulska-Hulme (2005) usability, an important key feature of m-learning, is characterised as "easy to learn, effective to use, efficient and enjoyable from the user's perspective" (Kukulska-Hulme 2005: 45). Kukulska-Hulme draws on a definition by Preece et al. (1994) to conclude that whether human-computer interaction will be rewarding is heavily intertwined with the concept of "user experience," which defines whether something is pleasing, and that in turn depends on user expectations, which "are shaped by the user's age, education, cultural background, gender and many other factors" (Kukulska-Hulme 2005: 45). Preece (2000, in Kukulska-Hulme 2005) makes the claim that "software with good usability supports rapid learning, high skill retention, low error rates and high productivity". From a pedagogical standpoint, the concept of usability entails "ensuring good educational experiences and enabling successful interactions" (Kukulska-Hulme 2005: 46). Yet another feature, not without significance for m-learners is "interoperability" (Hoppe 2006: 31), both of purely technical data exchange, cross platform use and information flow, as well as educational interoperability, i.e. adjusting to learning objectives.

The nature of m-learning embraces the interplay of concepts such as device functionality, mobility of the learner, formality/informality of the educational setting, fragmentation and bite-sized-ness of the educational experience, expectations regarding application usability, or technical and educational interoperability. It is also to a great extent context-sensitive and funnelled through affective factors such as, to begin with, attitudes and expectations towards the nature of human-device interaction (*Figure 9*).

*Figure 9: M-learning components matrix*

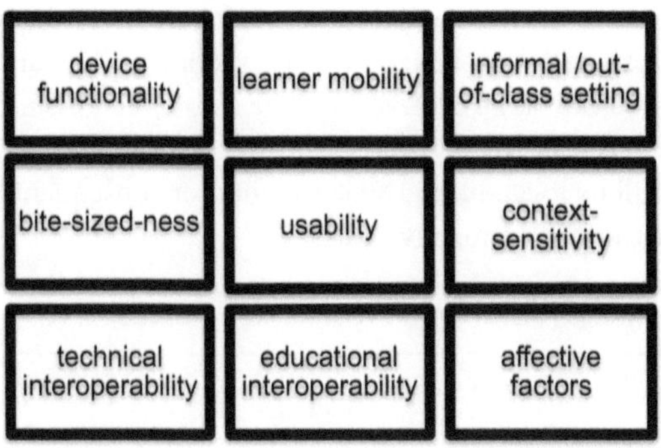


To conclude, m-learning has the capability to offer unique educational affordances due to the synergy emerging from features such as portability, social interactivity, context sensitivity, connectivity as well as individuality (see Klopfer et al. 2002). The following section will discuss intelligent flashcard vocabulary trainers as a possible software solution enabling such benefits.

## 4.5 Intelligent Vocabulary Trainers

With the growth of mobile technologies, developing technology-enhanced learning tools has become a critical issue in the field of ELT (Kukulska-Hulme – Traxler 2005: 180, Chen – Chung 2008). There have appeared numerous online vocabulary trainers designed to support personalized vocabulary learning. Highly elaborate algorithms have been used to facilitate memorization as well as to help integrate learning into one's daily routine, challenging the notion of what had been regarded as effective in pedagogic design (e.g. Cortez – Roy 2012). State-of-the-art online vocabulary trainers are more and more frequently enumerated in teacher training publications (Buttner 2007, Ma et al. 2013, Presson et al. 2013). These intelligent tutor systems are steadily becoming more popular (Stockwell 2007, in Kukulska-Hulme – Shield 2008: 274) as they allow personalized learner profiles to be created and deliver activities according to identified problem areas.

> "(…) everyday devices such as mobile phones can be highly effective and easier to adopt into practice, provided there is a good match between the technology and the learning that it is needed to support."
>
> (Kukulska-Hulme – Traxler 2005: 180)

Intelligent online tutors can be evaluated based on the content-based approach or the design-based approach. It seems that the future of mobile assisted language learning lies in The Language Partner software (Presson et al. 2013: 157). Such study tools should "run equally well on mobile devices and desktop computers", include "basic skills and vocabulary tutors, games, interactive media access, and situated learning activities" and "record student usage patterns and responses that will be logged into DataShop files for subsequent student modelling and linkage to classroom activities."

*Figure 10: The Language Partner (after Presson et al. 2013: 158)*

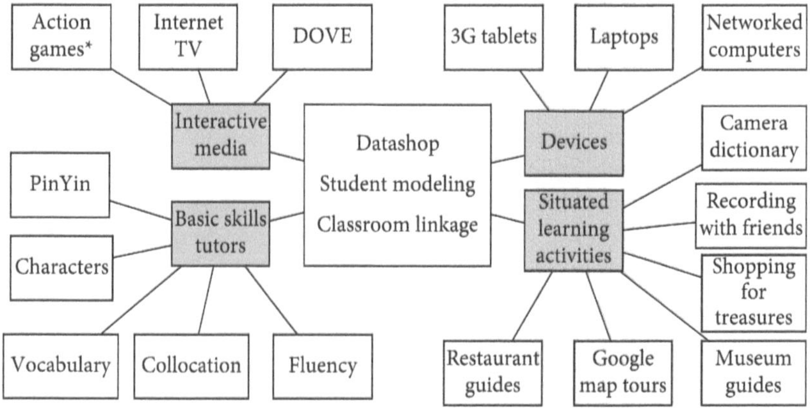


There are numerous design challenges that online vocabulary trainers need to face to be considered viable on hand held devices (Cortez – Roy 2012). Chen and Chung (2008) introduced a personalized mobile English vocabulary learning system based on item response theory (Baker 1992) and learning memory cycle. The system suggested appropriate vocabulary items for learning based on the individual learner's vocabulary ability and memory cycle. Their system was designed to be used on handheld mobile devices in such a way so as to maximize the efficiency of learning.

One of the key tenets of this system was its personalized learning scheme. First, the learner's vocabulary ability was assessed based on item response theory, and in the second stage the system recommended proper learning materials. Also, a vocabulary review module, adjusted for individual learners, was introduced. Based on the level of difficulty of a given item and individual learner's vocabulary ability, the system scheduled revision patterns so as to facilitate short term memory retention, but also to promote long term memory retention. In their article, Chen and Chung (2008) put a lot of emphasis on the system's architecture and its technological intricacies, computing vocabulary recommendation algorithms, vocabulary review process as well as the learning interface. Study results obtained by Chan and Chung (2008) confirmed that personalized mobile English vocabulary learning based on spaced repetition algorithms enhanced learner performance at a statistically significant level. Spaced-repetition software (SRS) enjoys great popularity and lies at the heart of the majority of online vocabulary learning tools which use flashcards. The next section encapsulates the key features of such learning tools.

## 4.6 Flashcard Software

With the first flashcards being introduced in the 19th century for phonics (Mortimer 1834), the technological developments of recent decades gave rise to digital flashcards and flashcard learning software. Flashcard software is an attempt to replace inefficient vocabulary lists and drills with a more interactive mode. Modern flashcard learning software allows the user to "integrate tools or games beyond a standard flashcard" (Buttner 2007: 1) enabling options such as embedded audio, visuals or monitoring progress.

Traditional flashcard learning was often based on the Leitner (1972) cardbox system, with graded flashcard mastery and items appearing for review at increasing time intervals. Most flashcard software algorithms also support this method of learning, as well as embrace Ebbinghouse's (1885) forgetting curve – see discussion in Pimsleur (1967), Landauer – Bjork (1978), Hulstijn (2001) or Randall (2007) – to optimize learning and decrease the time spent on building vocabulary.

There are numerous flashcard learning programs available. With new mobile apps mushrooming everyday, it seems impossible to present an up-to-date, complete list of flashcard software, nevertheless, I will briefly present some of the most popular flashcard systems from the perspective of their usefulness to the research project.

To the best of my knowledge, there are only a few independent efficacy studies on flashcard software interventions in learning English for Medical Purposes. Schmidmaier et al. (2011) investigated the use of electronic flashcards in medical education. The study demonstrated that repetitive testing is a potent learning strategy for short-term retention, but it did not confirm the efficacy of this method for long-term knowledge retention. In a randomized, controlled study, Taveira-Gomes et al. (2015) investigated spaced-repetition and test-enhanced recall accuracy among medical students using Alert Student, a spaced-repetition flashcard platform using test-enhanced learning. Bow et al. (2013) developed a crowdsourcing learning tool for medical students to share flashcards. Exam scores analysis revealed that the students who had access to the flashcard system outperformed those who did not. The above mentioned studies focused on medical content knowledge rather than language knowledge, therefore, it would be valuable to research the efficacy of flashcard spaced-repetition software in the context of learning English for Medical Purposes. For that reason one of the listed flashcard SRS programs would be chosen.

**Anki** (ankisrs.net) is a spaced repetition flashcard program using a modified SM2 algorithm. It enables adding user content and syncing on many devices via AnkiWeb. Among Anki's interesting features one can mention the text-to-speech module, learning statistics and the possibility to tag items for higher or lower priority, which affects the review schedule. Anki does not offer any gamification features, nor does the review scheme allow "on demand" review of a given item. The desktop version allows embedding of multimedia files. The Anki mobile app runs on both Android and iOS devices.

**Byki** (byki.com) learning software uses a spaced repetition flashcard interface with MP3 audio and learning games available in the upgraded mode. The system tracks learner progress, but although it runs on both Android and iOS devices, its free-of-charge version does not offer a course in English. Attractive as the software seems, it does not allow adding user content either.

**Cerego** (cerego.com) is an adaptive learning platform using a patented, spaced rehearsal method based on Ebbinghaus' forgetting curve. It offers features such as personalized learning experience, colour coding for Memory Permanence or detailed learning schedules. Cerego enables adding user content but it does not enable mobile learning on Android devices.

**CoboCards** (cobocards.com) is an online and mobile flashcard application. It enables adding content, offers control over the learning progress following the principles of Leitner's cardbox system. Nonetheless, it offers only two card sets free-of-charge.

**Course Hero** (coursehero.com) is an online learning platform to upload and compile study resources, e.g. course materials, flashcards, educational videos etc. Course Hero offers the interesting option of Optimal Learn – a flashcard management application allowing to set up deadlines for mastering a given data set. Course Hero offers only some of the courses free-of-charge. Also, the platform raises many copyright and plagiarism related controversies.

**Cram.com** (cram.com formerly **Flashcard Exchange**) is free, online flashcard learning software which offers over 119 million flashcards that can be learned by means of Jewels of Wisdom and Stellar Speller games to accompany study sets. However, the application does not support spaced repetition.

**Fresh Memory** (fresh-memory.com) is a spaced repetition flashcard application, similar to SuperMemo, based on the SM2 algorithm. Interestingly, this flashcard application offers "multiple sides" to each flashcard, which allows the creation of flashcard entries embracing a number of word uses. Fresh Memory does not run on mobile devices.

**Full Recall** (fullrecall.com) offers optimized, forgetting curve based, review schedules for flashcards. One of the more interesting features of the program is that the review algorithm is adjusted based on subjective learner estimates of the level of mastery of a given item – in contrast to other SRS systems which use objective effective recall estimates. Full Recall runs on Android devices and allows embedded images and sounds. It offers learning statistics and a "soft-limit" option that causes the revision of some items to be rescheduled for the following day if the system decides they can be postponed without much harm to the learning efficacy, i.e. some items are left for revision as obligatory today whereas the revision of others can be postponed until the next day.

**Goconqr** (goconqr.com previously **ExamTime**) is a learning platform that offers, among other things, creating flashcards that can be revised based on a spaced-repetition algorithm. The program supports visuals but not audio or multimedia. The ExamTime mobile app runs on iOS and Android devices.

**Gradint** (people.ds.cam.ac.uk/ssb22/gradint/) is a SRS learning tool following a modified Pimsleur (1967) language learning system. It enables creating sets of audio materials labelled "audio flashcards". **Gradint Web edition** offers a text-to-voice module, however, interesting as the idea of an "audio flashcard" may seem, in case of medical terminology, the prompts provided by the speech synthesizer are far from satisfactory, which in case of self-directed learning can lead to fossilization of incorrect pronunciation patterns.

**LearnThatWord** (learnthat.org) learning software was created in cooperation with the Open Dictionary of English database. The application uses spaced repetition and learner profile oriented quizzes. It supports video and audio but does not allow adding content. It is also limited to the ODE database, which makes it unsuitable for ESP learners.

**Memorang** (memorangapp.com) is a free spaced repetition learning platform offering multiple learning modes and a personalized learning experience. Designed to meet the needs of English-speaking medical students, the program offers a number of medical courses running on Android and iOS devices. Yet, because it focuses on content and not language knowledge, there is no text-to-speech or audio module.

**MemoryLifter** (memorylifter.com) is a spaced repetition flashcard system based on the Leitner (1972) box algorithm. It enables images, audio, video and offers a number of learning modes involving mnemonics and multi-sensory learning. The MemoryLifter network allows an educational experience in virtual learning groups. At the moment, the program offers eighty learning modules. It does not, however, run on mobile platforms.

The award-winning, online flashcard learning software, **Memrise** (memrise.com), uses mnemonics and spaced repetition. The gamified application enables managing student groups, creating courses, adding content and is said to adapt to personal learning styles. Memrise is supported by Android and iOS devices. A desktop version of Memrise allows embedding audio files, videos and images.

Launched in 2003, **Mnemosyne** (mnemosyne-proj.org) is a spaced repetition and spacing effect flashcard software using a modified SM2 algorithm. It attends to item difficulty. The application supports mobile phone learning. Designed as a research project on long-term memory retention (mnemosyne-proj.org/principles.php), the application collects data on the learning process.

**OpenCards** (opencards.info) is a learning tool offering PowerPoint (ppt-files) flashcard sets augmented with spaced repetition based on a SuperMemo scheduling algorithm. However, it does not support mobile phone learning, as cross-platform use is difficult due to syncing issues.

Launched in 2011, **Quizlet** (quizlet.com) is an online learning tool using flashcards, augmented with a text-to-speech module. Quizlet enables creating personalized study sets and managing student groups. Revision modes offer elements of gamification. It has both Android and iOS apps. However, it does not offer spaced repetition schemes.

**Pauker** (pauker.sourceforge.net) is a Java flashcard program using the Leitner cardfile system with **MiniPauker** offered for mobile devices. The program offers a simple flashcard editor, but does not support visuals or audio and does not display gamification elements.

**Repetitions** (repetitionsapp.com) is yet another spaced repetition system. It is a simple program offering cloud synchronization of study sets on multiple devices. The review algorithm is to a great extent based on a user self-assessment module. The program does not support visuals or audio.

Developed in the 1980s by the Polish researcher Piotr Woźniak, **SuperMemo** (supermemo.com), was the prototype for many flashcard programs. Although initially SuperMemo was not designed as language learning software, with time it became a trend setter among SRS. The latest versions of the program enable highly advanced formatting features and allow the use of multimedia as well as hypertexting. SuperMemo scheduling algorithms (see http://www.supermemo.com/english/algsm11.htm) are used by numerous flashcard applications. SuperMemo allows easily remembered items to be repeated less and less frequently, whereas items that are more difficult appear more frequently. It supports Android and iOS use. Released nearly quarter of a century ago, SuperMemo versions 1.0 to 16.0 have been widely researched by ELT and CALL specialists.

**Vocapp** (vocapp.com) uses multisensory flashcards and spaced repetition, and offers quizzes and self-assessment modules. It was developed by Polish researchers under a European Union grant for innovation. One of the advantages of Vocapp is its text-to-speech module as well as its multimedia database. Vocapp enables adding content but does not contain elements of gamification. It is supported by both Android and iOS devices.

**Voxy** (voxy.com) is a system of photo flashcards. It enables snapshots taken by the iPhone camera to be turned into digital flashcards augmented with a pronunciation module. Voxy's creators highlight the fact that this way of creating flashcards activates not only the visual but also the kinaesthetic mode, as well as contextual learning (real life objects). Voxy does not support spaced repetition, nor does it run on Android devices.

There are a number of features flashcard software needs to have to suit the needs of learners of English for Medical Purposes. Whereas General English courses offered on such platforms often do not need modification, the possibility to add content is an important feature from the point of view of an ESP practitioner, as ESP courses are always highly needs oriented. Also, in the case of English for Medical Purposes, the scope of specialist terminology is extensive and stretches beyond typical learner dictionaries. Moreover, creating flashcards can also be treated as an important part of the learning process.

Based on an overview of online flashcard software systems, the criteria for inclusion for flashcard software to be taken into account as a possible research tool were as follows: existence of a free-of-charge mode (premium charged versions might be available), non-proprietary mode (open-source materials), spaced repetition algorithm, supported by Android and iOS, offers elements of gamification, supports embedded visuals and audio, easy syncing and cross-platform use. In Chapter Five I discuss the effectiveness of mobile assisted learning of English for Medical Purposes using Memrise as an example of SRS with a web based, desktop platform as well as an easily synced mobile app to allow efficient use of handheld devices at the learner's convenience.

### 4.6.1 Memrise

Created by Ed Cooke and Greg Detre and launched in 2010, Memrise focuses on enhancing learning through scientifically optimized learning. The software uses the metaphor of "growing a garden of memory" by planting items in short term memory, harvesting them to long term memory and watering them in the review mode.

> "On Memrise, inspired by the organic nature of your memory, we've turned learning into a game where you grow a Garden of Memory. Every word begins life as a seed, you nurture it through reviews and tests until it grows strong, takes root and blossoms into a flower in your Long Term Memory (LTM). Once in Long Term Memory, you have to review each memory to keep it from fading – just like you'd water a flower to keep it healthy."
>
> (http://www.memrise.com/about/)

Though Memrise was designed as a playtime activity, the scientific component of Memrise (http://www.memrise.com/science/) involves: elaborate encoding, choreographed testing, and scheduled reminders. Among important features of Memrise Presson et al. (2013: 157) enumerate: gaming features, practice scheduling (based on spaced repetition) and encoding elaboration.

Elaborate encoding means integrating new knowledge to into the already existing memory framework to increase the likelihood of item retention, e.g. by means of association chains and creating mental images that bind items. An example provided by the Memrise creators is that of facilitating learning the word "aburrido" (boring) by creating a "mem" visualizing "it's boring to eat a burrito with every meal". As far as choreographed testing is concerned, Memrise's creators consider regular testing to be a powerful learning incentive and a way to promote long-term item retention through regular retrieval. Also, scheduled reminders are yet another Memrise feature that is supposed to boost learning efficacy. Review intervals are set up based on algorithms using Ebbinghaus' forgetting curve. Memrise allows eliminating words the learner considers as known, or words he/she is unwilling to learn, via the ignore button. An algorithm suggests the items to be reviewed, and items causing problems to the learner are revised more frequently, to facilitate short term retention as well as short to long term memory transfer. Memrise allows creating one's own mems and courses. The learning process is envisaged in the form of a leader board (which allows a teacher to keep track of student progress but also adds to the competitive edge). Among the strengths of Memrise, one might list its focus on effective time management (bite-sized practice in one's free time), mnemonics (a large pool of mems available, the possibility of creating personalized images) and intuitiveness of the software. One of the more frequently brought up disadvantages of Memrise, compared to other flashcard software, e.g. Vocapp or Quizlet, is the lack of a built-in pronunciation engine. Audio files need to be uploaded or recorded by the course designer. Also, courses often lack a difficulty curve, and beyond a mere "ignore" button for items already known, the program does not offer an interface to mark the degree of item mastery, unlike in, for example, Cerego or Full Recall. Compared to other flashcard software, e.g. Cram, LearnThatWord or Quizlet, Memrise's review mode offers a limited number of tasks, i.e. spelling exercises, word order exercises and multiple choice exercises, which make the revision mode monotonous and might discourage the learner. On the other hand, goal-setting interface options are an attempt to provide a sense of achievement and control over the learning process. Courses available on Memrise include not only user created content, but also courses delivered by Cambridge University Press, e.g. the Cambridge Upper-intermediate English course containing 1,000 words and phrases from Cambridge Dictionaries Online for English learners at the B2 level of language proficiency.

## 4.7 Technology in Teaching ESP

Following Robinson (1991, in Flowerdew 2013: 340) "(...) one would expect future ESP courses to adopt communication tools of the field, similar to the line of thinking that ESP courses should mirror the activities and methodologies employed in real-life ESP situations." The healthcare branch is quite effective in developing solutions for healthcare professionals, some of which can be used in EMP practice. As EMP is a well-established branch of ESP, (Hung et al. 2010: 255) there appear many useful websites or technological solutions that non-Anglophone speakers of EMP might benefit from, e.g. the Voice of America

News (voanews.com) website which provides health reports adjusted to the level of learners.

The General Medical Council (GMC) in the United Kingdom provides guidelines concerning good medical practice in the form of easily accessible interactive medical scenarios (gmc-uk.org/index.asp). From the point of view of an ESP practitioner, these interactive scenarios provide not only content, but also linguistic input. Learners can see what sort of language is used and which language forms are preferred in a given type of conversation, i.e. they can match language functions with real language use. Students find these types of exercises engaging as they (acting as virtual doctors) focus not only on content-related decisions and getting the message across, but also on passing it on to the patient using culturally appropriate forms.

In a recent project Loiacono (2013: 195–215) highlights the importance of exposure to various types of medical discourse, as well as developing an understanding of how discourse patterns influence every day healthcare practice. Loicano made a training film shot in a hospital surroundings that served as a model of interaction with which medical students whose mother tongue is not English can readily identify (Loiacono 2013: 196). The film was then cut into sequences, embedded in a website and additional exercises were added. Through means of, e.g. critical discourse analysis, learners are encouraged to reflect on sociomedical discourse. One of the major strengths of the project is that it appeals to non-native healthcare professionals. Loiacono highlights the importance of critical discourse analysis (CDA) of medical texts in view of teacher-learner interactions and presents a model of analysing healthcare texts. She suggests a new way of teaching medical English that would not focus on lexico-grammatical forms as "the sole objective" but one that puts emphasis on the sociomedical interaction of Genre, Text grammar and GMER (Global Minimum Essential Requirements in medical education) principles.

Following Johns and Price-Machado (2001: 52), it is becoming more and more important for ESP practitioners to run technology aided courses. Paltridge and Starfield (2013: 32) express a common view in the field that "(…) developments in technology are impacting on research and pedagogy in exciting ways towards a virtual learning environment".

ESP more and more often benefits from the use of corpora (see the discussion in Nesi 2013: 415–418), as it is not usually a domain-specifc terminology item that is the problem, but "the language that flanks it" (Coxhead 2013: 129). Corpus linguistics techniques can be of use in training programs to educate non-native healthcare professionals about EMP formulaic language, e.g. Adolphs et al.

(2004) *Applying Corpus Linguistics in a health care context,* Biber – Conrad (2004) *Corpus-Based Comparisons of Registers,* Skelton – Hobbs (1999) *Concordancing: the use of language-based research in medical communication,* Skelton et al. (2002) *'I' and 'we': a concordancing analysis of doctors and patients use first person pronouns in primary care consultations* or Thomas – Wilson (1996) *Methodologies for studying a corpus of doctor-patient interaction.* Lexical bundles or KWIC concordance lines (Key Word In Context concordance line, defined as node within a line of about 70 characters) are also often investigated by textbook writers to make informed decisions about relevant lexis and language patterns, e.g. *The Nottingham Health Communication Corpus* consists of more than 500,000 words from a variety of health care spoken and written contexts. For example, Skelton et al. (2002) examined doctor-patient consultations for the appearance of *as if, as though, look like and feel like* constructions. However, the most common way of exploring data provided by corpora is creating frequency based word lists. This is unfortunate, because according to Nesi (2013: 417) key word analysis or n-grams (lexical bundles), i.e. strings of words that frequently recur in a corpus, are more promising. Though, as Nesi (2013: 418–419) claims, although there is plenty of research on corpora, for various reasons individual ESP practitioners frequently do not look at that data.

## 4.8 Concluding Remarks

This chapter surveyed the current literature on mobile assisted learning, examining how it might be incorporated into the process of foreign language learning. Key points encapsulated the potential benefits of using mobile assisted language learning, as various studies have reported its positive impact on vocabulary learning and retention, and in particular that m-learning seems to be able to overcome the traditional temporal and spatial limits of the foreign language classroom. It has also shed light on the capabilities and possible constraints of implementing mobile technologies and flashcard vocabulary tutors in the process of learning and teaching English for Medical Purposes.

Although, on the pedagogical level, mobile learning is associated with informal educational contexts, with learners accessing learning materials "anytime, anywhere," there have been attempts to harness this kind of learning in institutionalised contexts. Based on the premise that mobile learning should be a part of a learning framework incorporating a variety of learning tools used in different contexts and "distributed over time and space," and guided by an assumption that there is not enough evidence to make claims about the efficacy of MALL (Kukulska-Hulme – Shield 2008: 280, Marcos et al. 2010), the research project discussed in Chapter Five is an attempt to provide hard data on the efficiency of MALL in the context of vocabulary learning in English for Medical Purposes.

The possible ways of incorporating mobile assisted language learning in a range of educational contexts requires further investigation, with special attention being placed on compliance with the principles of good teaching practice, as it is not about teaching with the use of technology but integrating technology into teaching practice, so that it can "support well grounded educational functions" (Hoppe 2006: 31). The latest m-learning definitions appropriately emphasize the role of the learner, rather than the role of technology and highlight the instrumental role of devices, and the need for MALL solutions to conform to second language pedagogy.

Despite the obvious limitations of flashcard learning systems, this way of learning does help develop metacognition by relating the new to the known, enabling personal experience and enhancing retrieval processes through scheduled practice. The research project undertaken was guided by the premise that spaced repetition software with in-built mnemonics can assist in memorisation of vocabulary and improve item retention. It must be highlighted that SRS is not understood as a comprehensive language learning tool but as a vehicle to achieve a threshold level of medical vocabulary that enables learning from context. SRS also gives learners a sense of control over the learning process though goal-setting interface options. One of the issues that requires further investigation is how best to overcome the limitations of flashcard systems, so that SRS systems could allow a truly self-directed, personalized educational experience.

In this discussion one also needs to take into account the fact that m-learning can successfully blur the line between personal and educational lives, which is in line with a psychological profile of "nomadic learners" (Alexander 2004) and the general assumption that only a fully mobile technology together with learners who are mobile when they learn will constitute a truly mobile educational activity for a "a new mobile conception of society" (Traxler 2005). Thus, the challenges education faces in the mobile age include not only technical problems and educational issues, but also social issues (Sharples 2006: 2).

Teachers should support learners in their endeavour to commence out-of-class student-initiated learning, as limited class time necessitates utilizing effective pedagogy, even if this means stepping out of the teacher comfort zone (see the discussion in Díaz-Vera 2012) and embracing the concept of, at worst, e-learning and at best u-learning (Rogers et al. 2005, Milrad 2006, Wilkerson et al. 2005), with m-learning being a middle of the road solution promoting handheld devices for self-paced language learning.

# Chapter Five: A Memrise-based Case Study

## 5.1 Introduction

Since, as has been discussed in the previous chapters, English is considered the language of science, there is a high degree of interest in the efficient teaching and learning of English for Medical Purposes to medical students. The following pages explore some of the critical questions arising from the attempts at translating theoretical insights into teaching English for Medical Purposes into actual practice. A further reason for undertaking the research was the my interest in mobile assisted learning of foreign languages, as well as the strong conviction that mobile phones should be considered as powerful educational devices. I investigated the process of expansion of the range of vocabulary in a group of first year medical students in collaboration with their English for Medical Purposes teacher. In an attempt to identify the issues in need of resolution and assess the proper scope of inquiry, I collected data both quantitative and qualitative in nature. In an attempt to segregate the questions in the study, I concentrated on the domains of learner motivation, digital literacy and attitude towards mobile assisted language learning as being those that open the way to the proper understanding of the vocabulary test results. Also, the research project contributed to the development of a handy inventory of medical terms and, hopefully, will contribute to the development of a mobile application for learning English tailored to the needs of medical students.

## 5.2 Research Goals

The study focused on the following research questions (RQs): RQ1: To what extent are medical students open to the use of (mobile)technology in learning English for Medical Purposes? RQ2: Can a self-paced Memrise-based homework enhance the learning of course material? RQ3: How do learners evaluate the Memrise-rooted MALL for EMP learning experience?

## 5.3 Research Method

### 5.3.1 Participants

A total of 40 first year medical students (25 women and 14 men) were asked to participate in the research project. Language instruction delivered to the study participants consisted of one 90-minute lesson of English for Medical Purposes per week. All students followed the same textbook and were taught by the same language teacher.

### 5.3.2 Research Instrument and Procedure

At the preliminary stage, the participants were asked to fill in an anonymous questionnaire (see Appendix A). Questionnaire 1 was distributed in Polish and comprised questions relating to: a) student motivation, knowledge of languages and learning preferences b) digital literacy and the use of technology in language learning and c) attitudes to m-learning. Data for the study were collected in the academic year 2014–2015. The study participants were then asked to sign up for Memrise and complete a course based on vocabulary sampled from Unit 3 from the textbook followed in the classroom. The reasons for choosing Memrise (an online flashcard SRS program) as the research tool were outlined in this book.

At this stage all the study participants were obliged to sign up for the course. Technical support was offered to any student requiring assistance in enrolling on the course, and throughout the project. The course mode was established as **obligatory** self-paced homework. The teacher monitored course attendance; however, when assigning the final grade she did not take into account the amount of points collected by the participants (which show the amount of material covered).

Having discussed Unit 3 in the classroom, the participants took an immediate vocabulary post-test and a delayed vocabulary post-test which was designed in such a way so as to constitute a part of the end of term test covering Units 1 to 3. This stage of the research project took place in the winter term of the academic year 2014–2015. The assumption was that having completed a Memrise-based course, the participants would be familiar with the program when entering the next stage of the research project, so that Memrise would not pose difficulty as a learning tool itself. Also, this design of the research project would help eliminate "the novelty factor" in Memrise usage.

The next stage of the research project involved self-paced Memrise-based homework in the form of a Memrise course based on vocabulary sampled from Unit 5 of the textbook followed in the classroom. However, this time the course mode was changed to **voluntary** self-paced homework. Students were offered an opportunity to enrol on the course after completing a vocabulary pre-test. Then, Unit 5 content was discussed in the classroom and followed by a vocabulary post-test. This stage of the research project took place in the spring term of the academic year 2014–2015.

In the final stage, the participants were asked to fill in an anonymous post-project questionnaire (see Appendix B). Questionnaire 2 was distributed in Polish and comprised questions relating to: a) learning time and learning device preferences b) evaluating Memrise as a learning tool and c) post-project attitudes to m-learning.

Statistical analysis of student responses was performed by means of the *IBM SPSS* version 20 for Windows and involved both questionnaire data and vocabulary test results.

## 5.4 Group Profile

### 5.4.1 Group Characteristics

In order to gain insight into the group profile of the study's participants the following variables were analyzed: gender, motivation to study medicine, knowledge of foreign languages, motivation to learn English for Medical Purposes, time spent leaning English for Medical Purposes and convictions about what constitutes success in learning a foreign language.

The reason behind investigating the patterns of medical students' motivation early in the undergraduate programme was to identify and examine the possible factors relevant to learning English for Medical Purposes. The participants of the study were asked to describe their motivation for choosing a career in medicine. Most participants chose more than one answer to this question. The results are shown in *Figure 11*.

*Figure 11: Why did you choose to study medicine?*

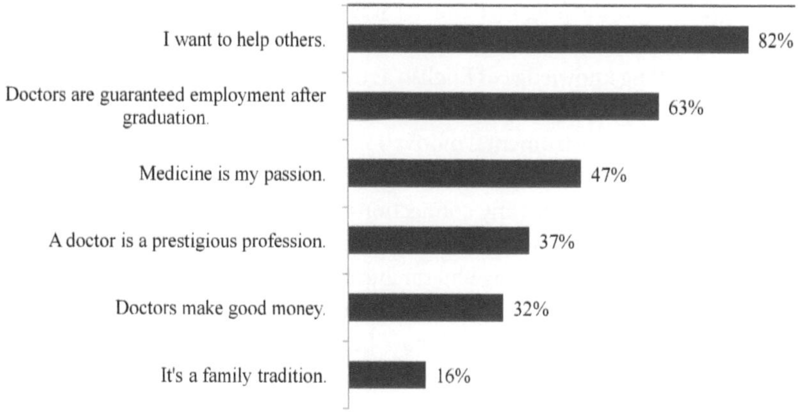

As *Figure 11* shows, two types of motives ranked high on intensity. The study participants pointed both to intrinsic motivation and internally generated motives (e.g. *I want to help others, Medicine is my passion*) and extrinsic motivation and externally generated motives (e.g. *Doctors are guaranteed employment after graduation, Doctors make good money*). Nearly half of the study participants declared a genuine interest in medicine itself. Both types of motivation for choosing a career in medicine were prominent among the participants of the study. I also investigated the motivation for learning English for Medical Purposes. The results are listed in *Figure 12*.

*Figure 12: What motivates you to learn English for Medical Purposes?*

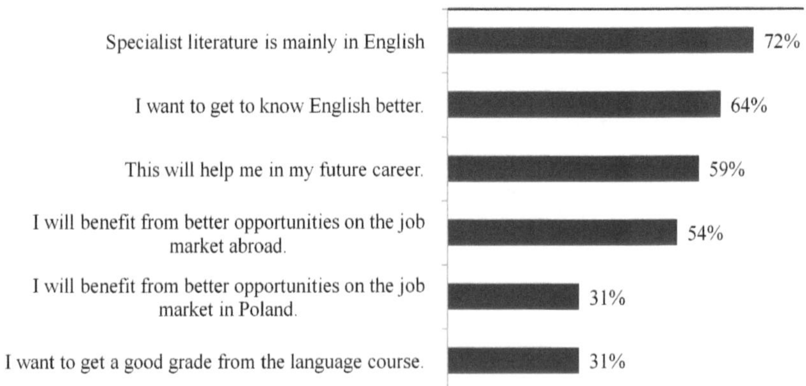


The results showed that short-term instrumental motivation (e.g. *I want to get a good grade from the language course*) was quite low on the scale. The study participants seemed to be well aware of the fact that that their future profession requires a working knowledge of English as the language of science (e.g. *Specialist literature is mainly in English*) and a vehicle for professional communication, i.e. denoting long-term instrumental motivation. Integrative motivation in the form of genuine interest in the English language ranked second.

To examine if there were any connections between particular motivations to learn English for Medical Purposes, a hierarchical analysis of variables was calculated (between-groups linkage hierarchical clustering and squared Euclidean distance for distance measure). The results show that two separate types of motivation could be distinguished, which have been labelled *specific* and *general*. The specific motivation was connected with the students' current goals: grade from the course and future employment. The general motivation was oriented on a better knowledge of English, which was related to reading specialist literature (see *Figure 13*) but indirectly also with the notion of self-development and life-long learning.

*Figure 13: Dendrogram of student motivation to learn English for Medical Purposes*

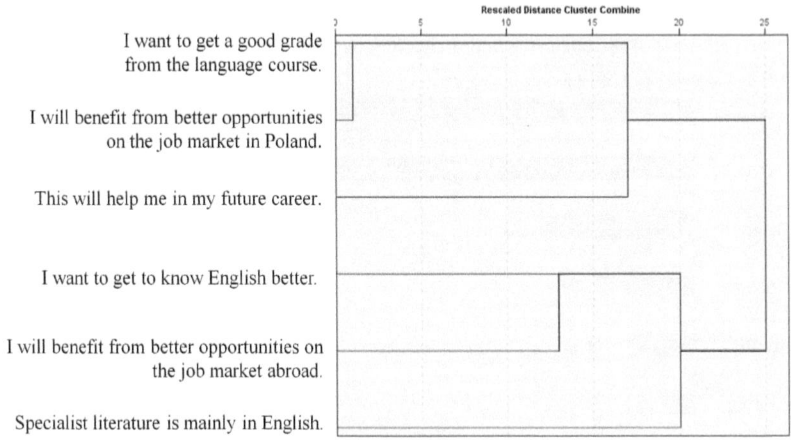


To obtain a more detailed motivational profile, the study participants were also asked about the sources of success in learning a foreign language. The results are shown in *Figure 14*.

*Figure 14: Factors influencing success in foreign language learning*

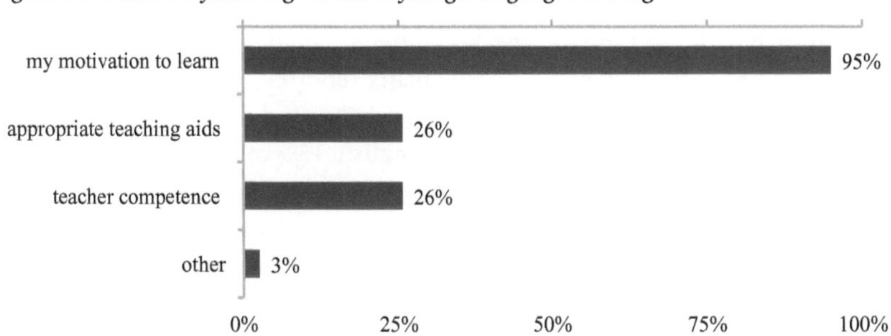


Student responses clearly lent support to the claim that for them personal/internal motivation was the driving force behind success in learning a foreign language (95%). Surprisingly, teacher competence was considered as the most important factor only by approximately one fourth of the study participants (26%) and was considered equally important, or equally unimportant, as teaching aids (26%).

These findings are interesting in the light of the discussion on teacher competence in English for Specific Purposes earlier in this book.

I was also interested in the number of foreign languages the study participants spoke, other than English. The results are presented in *Figure 15.*

*Figure 15: Apart from English, what foreign languages do you know?*

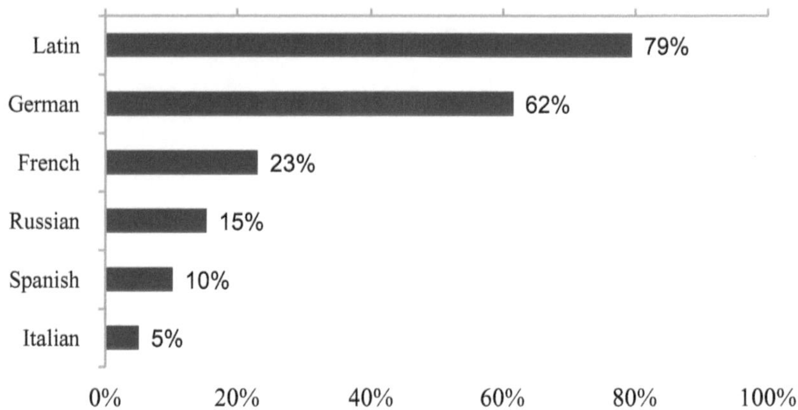


The participants reported a knowledge of Latin (79%), German (62%), French (23%), Russian (15%), Spanish (10%) and Italian (5%). Three participants reported the knowledge of other languages: Lithuanian (1 person), Japanese (1 person) and Ukrainian (1 person).

Latin included, the ratio for speaking foreign languages other than English was as follows: 54% of the study participants reported the knowledge of two foreign languages other than English, 18% of the study participants reported speaking one foreign language other than English, 15% of the study participants reported speaking three foreign languages other than English, 5% of the study participants reported speaking four foreign languages other than English and 3% (1 student) of the study participants reported speaking five foreign languages other than English. Two study participants reported the knowledge of English only. The results are shown in *Figure 16.*

*Figure 16: The knowledge of foreign languages other than English (Latin included)*

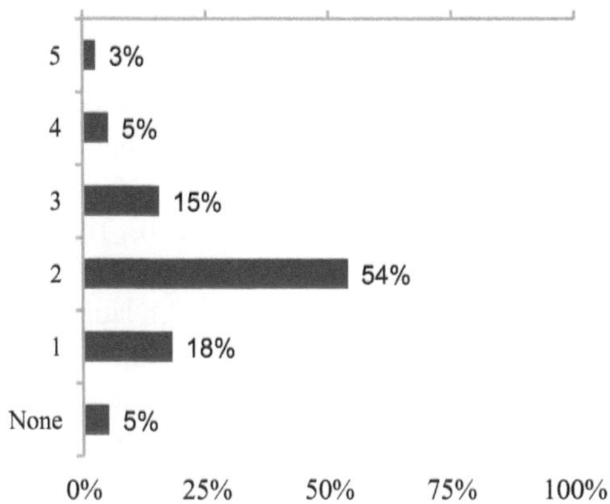


Latin excluded, the ratio for speaking foreign languages other than English was as follows: 64% of the study participants reported the knowledge of one foreign language other than English, 13% of the study participants reported speaking two foreign languages other than English and the same number of study participants reported not knowing any foreign language other than English, 5% (2 students) reported knowing three foreign languages other than English and the same number of study participants reported speaking four foreign languages other than English. The results are shown in *Figure 17*.

*Figure 17: The knowledge of foreign languages other than English (Latin excluded)*

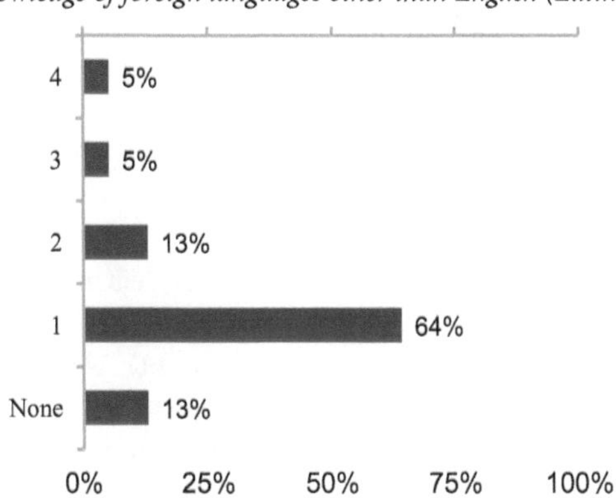


On the basis of the results illustrated in *Figures 16* and *17* (Latin included/Latin excluded), it can be concluded that the study participants had considerable experience as learners/users of foreign languages, and that this experience might have had an influence on the way they learnt English for Medical Purposes.

To investigate this issue, the study participants were asked whether and how, in their opinion, speaking foreign languages helped them learn English for Medical Purposes. Unsurprisingly, most of the study participants pointed to the knowledge of Latin as a factor facilitating learning English for Medical Purposes (more about the role of Latin in EMP in Chapter Two). They recognized the usefulness of knowing Latin in learning word stems and medical terminology. None of the study participants directly pointed to a foreign language other than Latin.

As far as time spent learning English is concerned, the majority of the study participants reported spending no more than one hour a week learning English in their free time (69%) and nearly four times as few study participants spent one to two hours doing so. Less than 8% of the study participants learnt English for two to three hours and slightly above 5% of the study participants spent more than three hours learning English. The results are presented in *Figure 18*.

*Figure 18: Apart from regular classes, how much time do you spend learning English for Medical Purposes?*

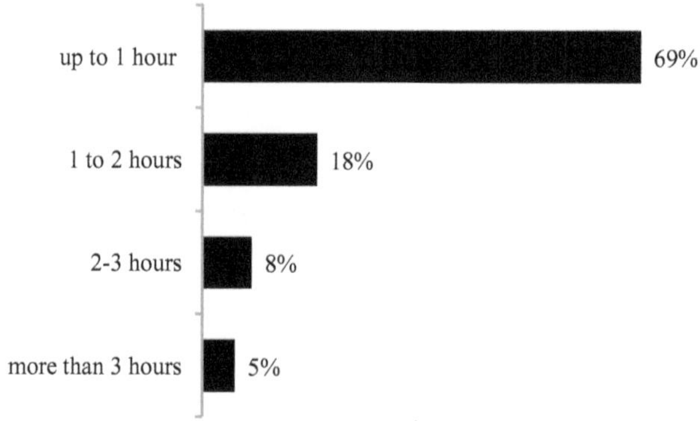


When inquired about the exact time of day when learning English, the study participants reported doing so at all times of the day (24% in the morning, 13% in the afternoon, 46% in the evening, 26% at night). Nearly one-third of the study participants (31%) indicated studying English when commuting to and from the university. Also, many study participants hinted at studying English simultaneously with other classes at university and while learning anatomy or other medical subjects.

### 5.4.2 Concluding Remarks

The emerging picture shows a group of young people with mixed motivation orientation towards both studying medicine and learning English for Medical Purposes. In general, they spend up to one hour learning English in various contexts, e.g. when commuting and at various times of the day, sometimes using English as a vehicle for learning content knowledge. They speak at least two foreign languages and are convinced that their motivation is a key factor in successful foreign language learning. Therefore, it would be interesting to investigate whether such a group would readily take up the challenge of self-paced mobile-enhanced homework containing elements of gamification.

## 5.5 Statistical Analysis of Research Questions

### 5.5.1 Answer to Research Question 1: To what extent are medical students open to the use of (mobile) technology in learning English for Medical Purposes?

To provide an answer to Research Question 1, the following questions concerning digital literacy from Questionnaire 1 were analyzed: *Which of the following devices do you have? How often do you use social networks (Facebook, Twitter, Instagram, etc.)? How often do you use a phone/smartphone to use the Internet? How do you access the internet/web content on your mobile phone?*

*Figure 19* illustrates the ownership of digital devices among the study's participants, while *Figure 20* illustrates the number of devices owned. Among the devices listed, 36% of the study participants owned two devices, 31% of the study participants owned three devices, 26% of the study participants owned four devices and two study participants owned as many as five devices. What needs to be highlighted is that the results show that there was one student who did not have a smartphone (though she had a laptop), which is congruent with the results obtained in the open questions section.

*Figure 19: The ownership of digital devices among the study participants*

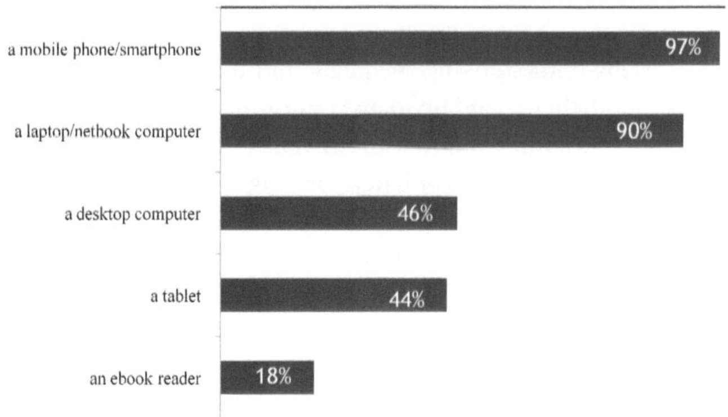


The fact that the study participants owned a number of digital devices suggests that the issue of cross platform use of a learning application, and thus synchronizing the course material covered on one device with course content accessed via other devices would be of importance as a feature of a mobile learning application.

*Figure 20: The number of digital devices owned*

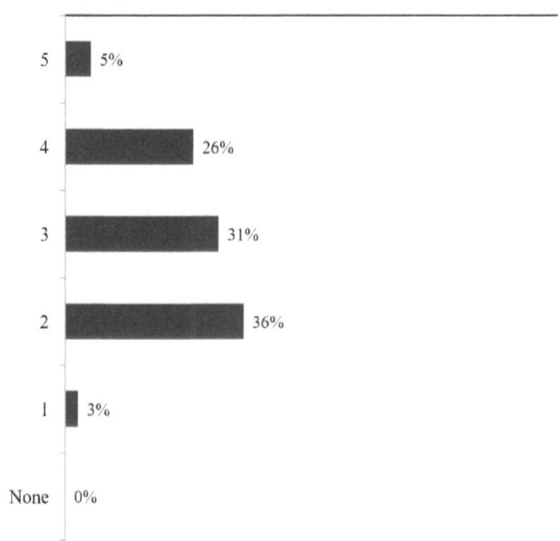


All study participants who filled in Questionnaire 1 reported the use of social networks/media, e.g. Facebook, Twiter, Instagram etc. The majority of the study participants reported connecting to social networks many times a day (67%),

17.9% of participants indicated being constantly logged in and 13% of the study participants would do it once daily. Only one student reported connecting to social networks as rarely as 2–3 times a week. The results are presented in *Figure 21.*

*Figure 21: Frequency of use of social networks*

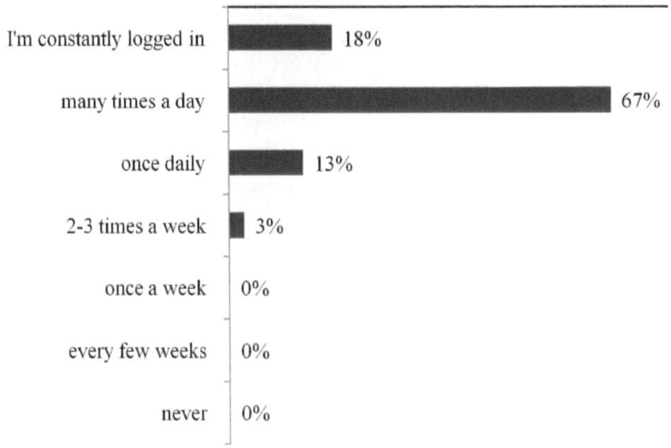


The study participants reported the following frequency of the use of a mobile phone/smartphone to connect to the Internet: the majority of the study's participants have access to web content many times a day (67%) and 15% are constantly logged in. Approximately 5% of participants use a mobile phone to access web content once daily, once a week and every few weeks, and one student does not use a mobile phone to access web content at all. The results are presented in *Figure 22.*

*Figure 22: How often do you use a mobile phone/smartphone to use the Internet?*

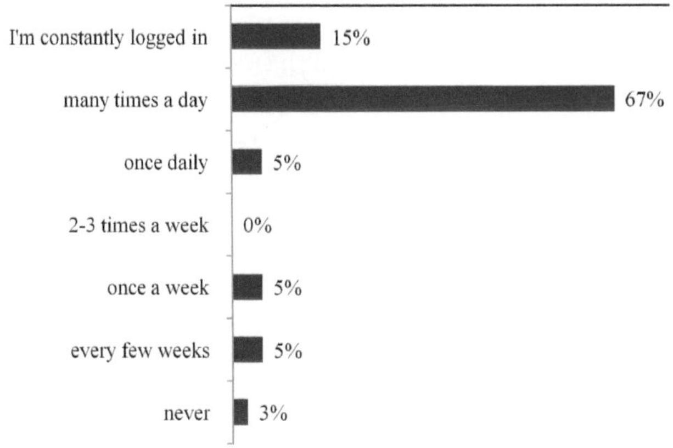

The study participants (n=39) reported the following means of accessing web content on their mobile phones: limited data transfer leading to the use of free wifi whenever possible – 56%, unlimited data transfer – 21%, only free wifi – 18% and no access to the internet via a mobile phone due to the costs – 5%. A combination of the frequency of accessing web content and the cost factor when doing so points to the premise that offline use might rank highly among the desired features of a mobile learning app. The results are presented in *Figure 23*.

*Figure 23: How do you access web content on your mobile phone?*

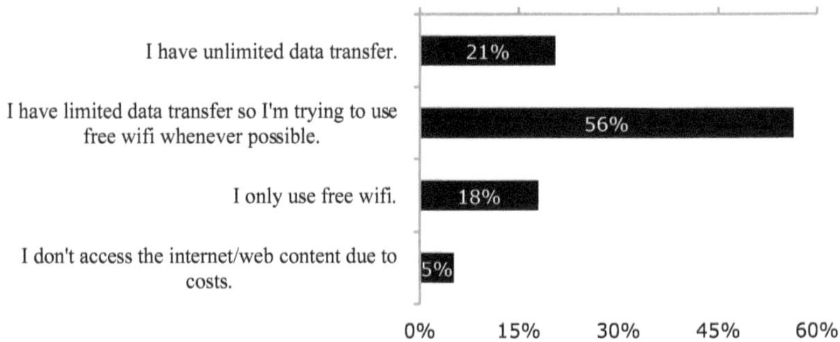


Apart from issues related to digital literacy, the study participants were also asked a number of questions regarding the use of technology in language learning. The questions were as follows: *Which devices do you use to learn English? And how often? Do you use any particular websites/educational platforms to learn English? If yes, which ones? If not, why not? Have you ever used any particular computer software to learn English? If yes, which one? If not, why not? Have you ever used any mobile apps to learn English? If yes, which ones? If not, why not? Would you be interested in learning English for Medical Purposes via a mobile app?*

As far as the devices used to learn English and the frequency of their use are concerned, none of the study participants reported daily use of a desktop computer or daily use of a tablet. One student reported daily use of a laptop/netbook (3%) and one student reported daily use of a smartphone (3%). Approximately one-third of study participants reported frequent use of a laptop/netbook and 13% of the study participants reported frequent use of a desktop computer. Surprisingly, although 44% of the study participants owned tablets (see *Figure 19*) only one study participant reported frequent use of a tablet to learn English. As many as 21% of the study participants declared frequent use of a mobile phone to learn English, and as many as 49% of the study participants openly declared rare use of a mobile phone to learn English. The results are presented in *Figure 24*.

On the other hand, in the open question section of Questionnaire 1 a number of the study participants openly reported a lack of knowledge about mobile assisted language learning, which might partly explain the rare use of a mobile phone as an educational tool.

*Figure 24: Which devices do you use to learn English? And how often?*

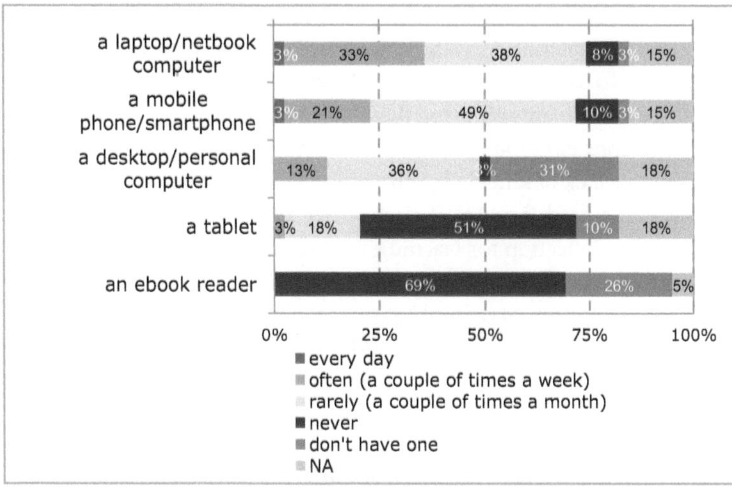


When asked about the use of websites/learning platforms for EFL, the study participants mostly reported the broadly understood *use of the Internet* and rather infrequent use of online dictionaries. Among educational tools used by the study's participants (both for computer and mobile use) were: Cambridge Dictionary (dictionary.cambridge.org), BBC Learning English (bbclearningenglish.com), Busuu (busuu.com), Google/Google Translate (translate.google.pl), Getionary (getionary.pl), eTutor (etutor.pl), BBC Radio (bbc.co.uk/radio), Ororo.tv (ororo.tv), Quizlet (quizlet.com), Dictionary.com (dictionary.reference.com), Leksyka.pl (leksyka.pl), Duolingo (duolingo.com), a website for mobile applications for learning foreign languages (uczsiejezyka.pl/aplikacje-mobilne-jezyki), flashcard software at pl.bab.la (pl.bab.la) and Anki (ankisrs.net). None of the study participants specifically mentioned the use of Memrise as an educational tool.

As reasons for not using educational platforms, the study participants enumerated: lack of time, preference for traditional/pen-and-pencil materials and textbooks, no need to use educational platforms, lack of software, lack of knowledge about educational platforms or satisfactory educational software, regarding course materials as sufficient, dissatisfaction with software/platform used, unwillingness to learn via computer enhanced methods and the cost factor. One participant openly criticized learning English via computer software.

When asked about the use of mobile applications for EFL, the majority of the participants reported not using mobile devices. Generally speaking, the reasons indicated by the participants did not substantially differ from those that prevented them from using learning platforms or computer software and encompassed: lack of time, preference for traditional/pen-and-pencil materials and textbooks, regarding course materials as sufficient, lack of opportunity to use mobile apps, having no need to use an educational platform and the cost factor. What differed was that three participants reported that their mobile phones did not support the use of mobile apps either at all or at a satisfactory level. The study participants also pointed to a lack of knowledge about useful applications and dissatisfaction with applications used (i.e. ANKI flashcards). Only two students reported the use of a mobile application for learning English for Medical Purposes (a mobile application for learning anatomy, medical flashcards), yet they did not specify the name of the application or applications.

The vast majority of students declared they would be interested in learning English for Medical Purposes via a mobile application. Five out of 39 students were against learning English this way. The results are shown in *Figure 25*.

*Figure 25: Would you be interested in learning EMP via a mobile app?*

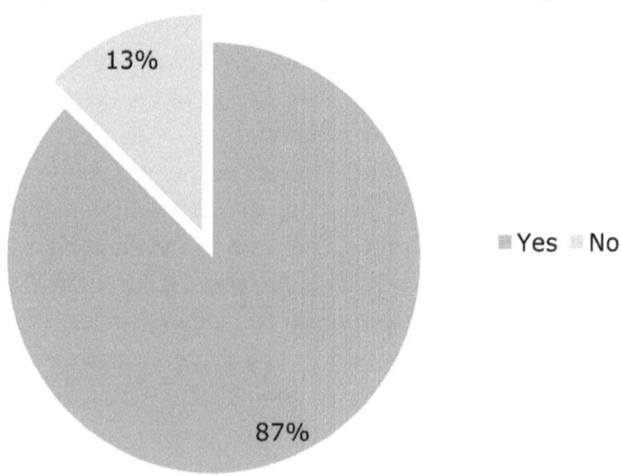


To sum up, for whatever reason, the participants of the study were not very au fait with mobile learning. Thus, in the first stage (Unit 3), the use of Memrise was obligatory so that all participants would get to know the learning tool. This way, in the second stage (Unit 5) the novelty factor, the knowledge of the program or technical issues would not play such a crucial role.

Yet another step to provide an answer to Research Question 1 was the analysis of the following questions concerning attitudes towards m-learning from Questionnaire 1: *Which 3 features of a mobile learning app do you think are most important? Grade the following statements: Mobile learning makes learning personalized. / Mobile learning is convenient and effective way of learning. / In the future, mobile learning will play an important role in English language learning. / Mobile learning is not an effective way of learning. / Mobile devices can be a good supplementation of a language course. / Mobile devices are easy to use. / A mobile phone is a convenient tool to learn English for Medical Purposes. / I'm willing to pay for access to a mobile learning platform. / I prefer mobile devices to a desktop computer.*

The list of desired features of a mobile application obtained in Questionnaire 1, before any of the study participants signed up for Memrise, is presented in *Figure 26.* As mentioned in the section on group characteristics and digital literacy, the cost factor and the possibility of offline use ranked highly among the study participants. Conversely, cross platform use was important only to 21% of the study participants. This might have been the case due to the fact that the study participants were asked to choose only the three most important features. The results are presented in *Figure 26.*

*Figure 26: Which three features of a mobile learning app do you think are most important?*

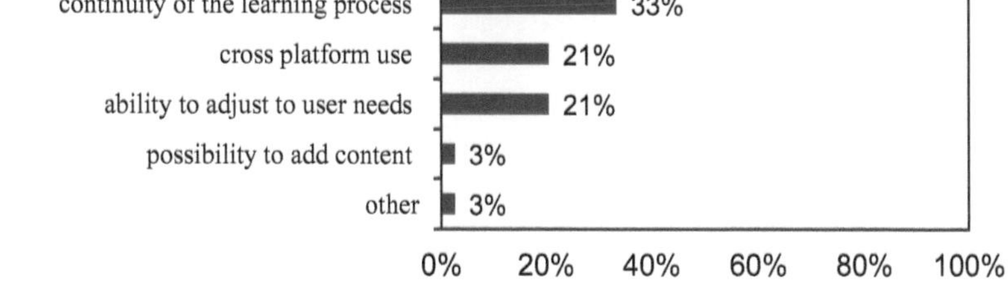


To examine how these various features of a mobile learning app are related with each other, a hierarchical analysis of variables was calculated (between-groups hierarchical clustering and squared Euclidean distance as a distance measure). On the grounds of the results (see *Figure 27*) three main clusters of app features were distinguished: personalization of the learning process, usage simplicity, cost.

The first cluster is related to personalization of the learning process, which is related to process continuity, but also the possibility of adding content. The second branch is composed of various elements relating to usage simplicity, i.e. possibility of use across various platforms, but also adjusting the application to user needs. The third branch comprises offline usage and price. It might be assumed that willingness to pay for the application, or rather the lack of it, reflects a general tendency of using only free of charge applications. On the other hand, as offline usage can be directly linked to the cost factor (the cost of data transfer) and many students reported a lack of unlimited data transfer and using free wifi as the main source of internet access, the cost factor does seem to play a role in the student population.

It should also be pointed out that as far as the first two branches, i.e. personalization and simplicity, are somehow related, the latter one, i.e. cost is visibly a separate factor, notably because both the cost factor and offline use were mentioned by about three out of four students. This means these features are the most important ones, but it could also mean students are not ready to pay for personalization of an application or simplicity of use.

*Figure 27: Dendrogram of the most important features of a learning mobile app*

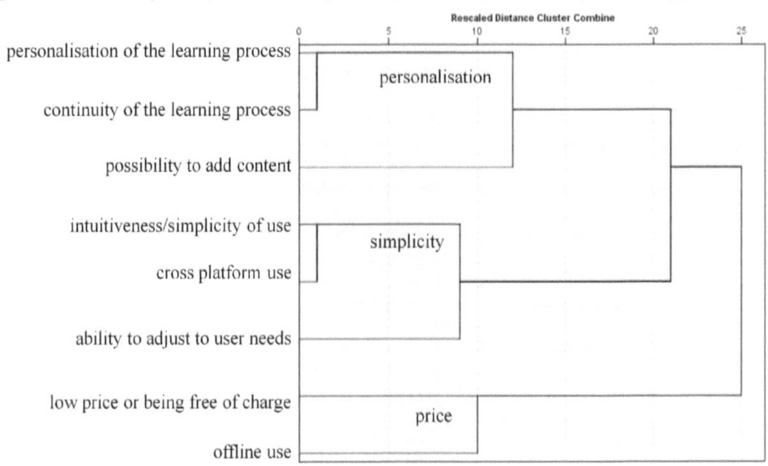


This analysis can be further illustrated by the detailed results of the Questionnaire 1 items relating to students attitudes towards m-learning which were assessed before the study participants signed up for Memrise. The results are given in *Figures 28 to 35.*

*Figure 28: Mobile learning makes learning personalized*

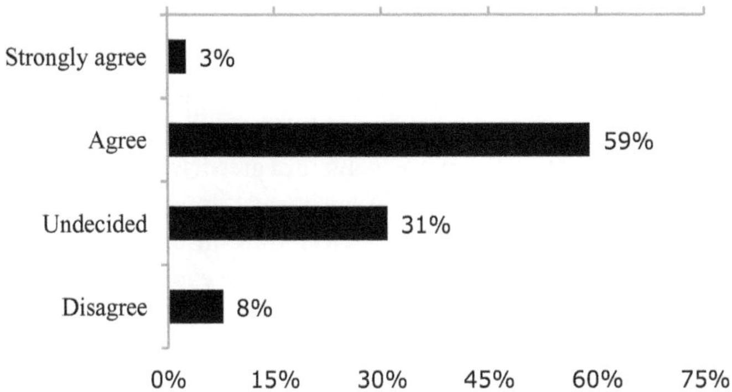


As can be seen in *Figure 28*, at baseline, the majority of the study participants (59%) were quite convinced that mobile learning makes the learning process personalized. Nearly 3% of the study participants strongly supported that view and none of the participants strongly disagreed with it. Almost 31% of the study participants did not have a clear view on the matter and 8% of study participants disagreed with the statement.

*Figure 29: M-learning is a convenient and efficient way of learning*

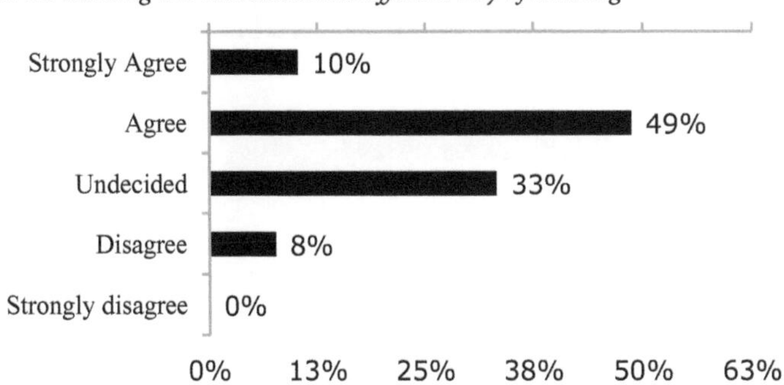


As demonstrated above, 49% of the study participants considered m-learning efficient, even though, as discussed on the preceding pages, the group could not be described as adept at m-learning. The 10% of the study participants who strongly agreed with the statement and the 8% percent of the participants who disagreed with it would probably encompass those students who also reported frequent use of educational software/applications, or disappointment with the software/applications used. Approximately one third of the study participants did not have a clear view on the matter, therefore it would be interesting to see if their opinions changed after completing the research project.

It might be assumed that in the age of digitalization, the study participants, who are young people, would support the claim that in the future m-learning will play an important role in learning English. However, the results were not unanimous here. None of the participants disagreed with the claim, slightly above 20% of participants were strongly convinced this would be so, 51% agreed with the claim and 28% did not have a clear view on the matter. It would be interesting to investigate whether those students who expressed a preference for the traditional/pen-and-paper way of learning, or even dissatisfaction with m-learning, acknowledge that m-learning will be dominant in the future, despite the fact that it is not their preferred way of learning but a general tendency that cannot be stopped.

*Figure 30: In the future, mobile learning will play an important role in English language learning*

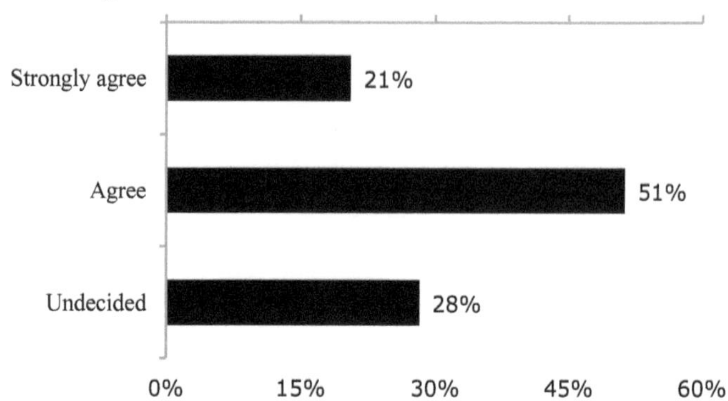


As far as course material supplementation was concerned, in the open questions a number of study participants pointed to the fact that they considered the materials provided during the language course to be sufficient. Most study participants agreed, or strongly agreed (53% and 40%, respectively) that m-learning might provide a good supplementation to a language course. Two students did not have a clear view on the matter and one student strongly disagreed. It can be concluded that the participants were initially open to the idea of course supplementation with mobile assisted language learning.

*Figure 31: Mobile devices can be a good supplementation of a language course*

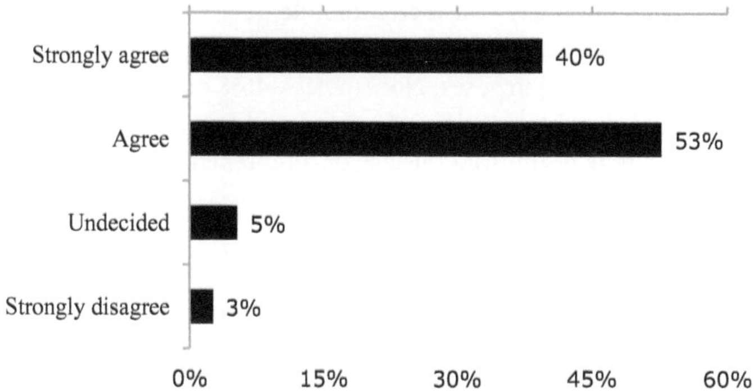


A total of 51% of students strongly agreed that mobile phones were easy to use and one-third of students agreed with this statement, therefore this notion should not be an obstacle to using Memrise via a mobile device. Especially that 46% of the participants declared that a mobile phone is a convenient device to learn English for Medical Purposes with. 18% of the participants strongly supported the claim and 28% were undecided. Again, 5% of the study participants (2 students) strongly disagreed, which might suggest that there was a small group of students who did not enjoy using mobile devices in general, which extended to learning via mobile devices as well. It is worth recalling at this point that three students reported that their mobile phones did not support the use of mobile applications, so this group of students would probably disagree with the claim on technical and not ideological grounds.

*Figure 32: Mobile devices are easy to use*

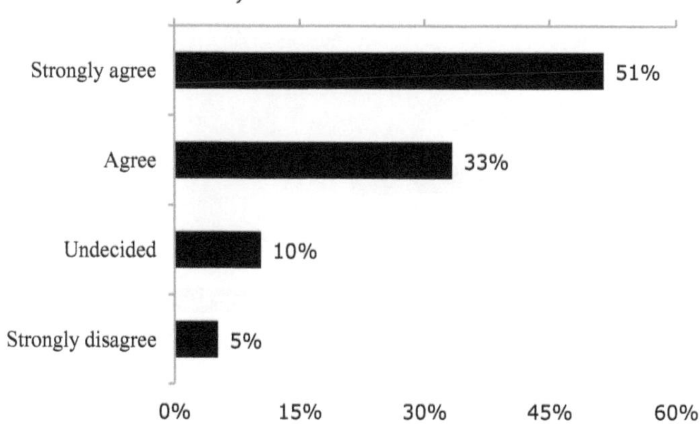

At this point it seems important to highlight that while as many as 51% of the study participants definitely considered mobile devices easy to use, only 18% strongly supported the claim that mobile devices are convenient tools for learning English for Medical Purposes. Nonetheless, 46% of the study participants supported the claim and as many as 28% of the study participants did not have a clear view, which may result from the lack of comprehensive or sufficient MALL learning experience.

*Figure 33: A mobile phone is a convenient tool to learn English for Medical Purposes*

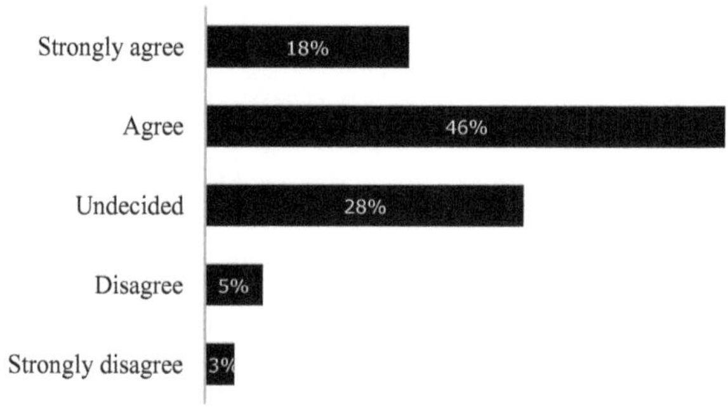


As far as the cost factor is concerned, only approximately 18% of the participants were willing to pay for access/subscription to a mobile learning platform. One student would definitely do so. Nearly 13% of the study participants were undecided and 67% of the study participants would not pay for such a subscription. It would be interesting to investigate whether this tendency stems purely from the cost factor, or rather the general tendency to use only free mobile applications, or a combination of both.

*Figure 34: I'm willing to pay for access to a mobile learning platform*

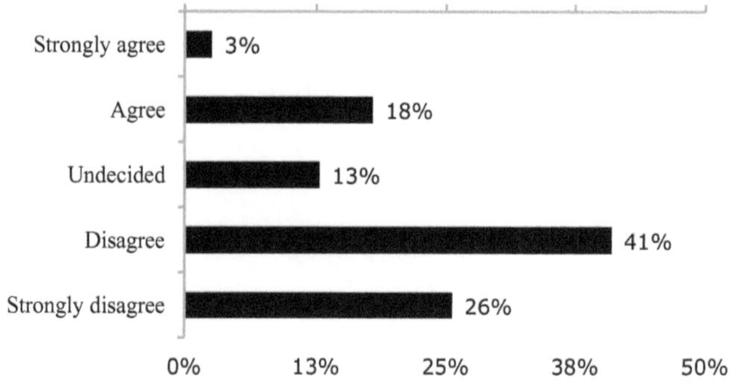

When referring to convenience, 51% of the participants stated that they preferred mobile devices to a desktop computer, 18% stated the contrary and nearly 31% were undecided.

*Figure 35: I prefer mobile devices to a desktop computer*

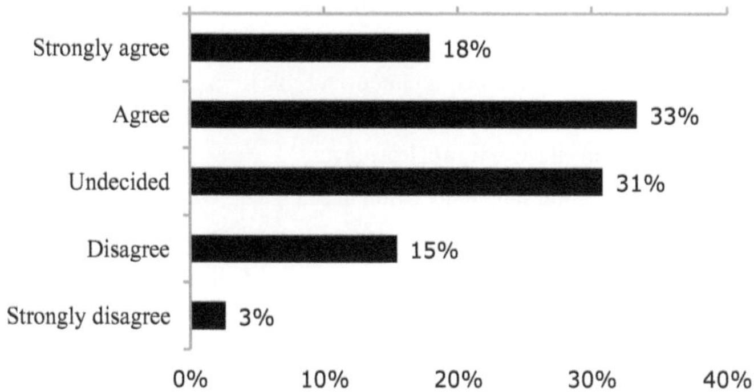


To examine student attitudes towards mobile learning, a Principal Component Analysis of nine Likert scale statements was performed. The results show three components which could be identified as: Effectiveness (factor 1), Simplicity (factor 2), Price (factor 3).

As for Effectiveness, statements such as: *Mobile learning is a convenient and effective way of learning, Mobile learning is not an effective way of learning* and *In the future, mobile learning will play an important role in English language learning* had the highest absolute loading (all loading above 0.7). The Simplicity component comprised statements such as *Mobile devices are easy to use, I prefer mobile devices to a desktop computer*, and *A mobile phone is a convenient tool to learn English in Medicine*. The Price component encompassed statements: *I'm willing to pay for access to a mobile learning platform* and – with negative loading – *Mobile devices can be a good supplementation of a language course.*

The statement about personalization of learning had a similar and high loading in both Effectiveness and Simplicity, so it should not be taken into account in any of them. The components emerging from this analysis are very similar to the branches indicating the most important features of a learning mobile app (see *Figure 16*). Therefore, it might be assumed that if there were more statements about personalization, it would become a component on its own, while Effectiveness and Simplicity would become components of a bigger meta-factor. In the light of the above, the author is planning further research on personalization as a driving force behind success in mobile learning.

*Table 12: Attitudes towards mobile learning – Rotated Component Matrix (Varimax)*

| | **Factor** | | |
|---|---|---|---|
| | **1** | **2** | **3** |
| Mobile learning makes learning personalized. | .475 | .397 | |
| Mobile learning is a convenient and efficient/effective way of learning | .796 | | |
| In the future, mobile learning will play an important role in English language learning. | .705 | | |
| Mobile learning is not an effective way of learning. | -.741 | | |
| Mobile devices can be a good supplementation of a language course. | .584 | | -.609 |
| Mobile devices are easy to use. | | .782 | |
| A mobile phone is a convenient tool to learn English for Medical Purposes. | .638 | .623 | |
| I'm willing to pay for access to a mobile learning platform. | .346 | | .839 |
| I prefer mobile devices to a desktop computer. | | .769 | |

The occurrence of the price factor in both the dendrogram and the factor matrix might suggest that most students are either not ready to pay for a mobile learning application, or they have not come across a product they would be willing to pay for.

### 5.5.2 Answer to Research Question 2: Can self-paced Memrise-based homework enhance the acquisition of course material?

To provide an answer to Research Question 2, the author conducted a multilayer analysis and analyzed the following questions from Questionnaire 2: *Did you use Memrise to learn vocabulary from Unit 5? If not, why? How much time did you spend on learning using Memrise? When did you use Memrise most often?*

#### *5.5.2.1 The Analysis*

The analysis consisted of several stages. As a preliminary step in the analysis of the results, progress, or the lack of it, in the learning of course content was examined by comparing the results of a Unit 5 pre-test with the results of a post-test administered after Unit 5. For that reason a paired sample one-tailed directional t-test was used. The t value (-2.41) showed that the mean in the post-test (22.9) was significantly higher ($p<0.01$, $df=39$) than the mean in the pre-test (10.45). The results shown in *Table 13* lent considerable support to the idea that the process of learning was effective.

*Table 13: Mean equality test*

| | Mean | N | t | p (one-tailed) |
|---|---|---|---|---|
| U5 pre-test | 10.45 | 40 | -2.41 | .01 |
| U5 post-test | 22.90 | 40 | | |

The second question was did the use of Memrise affect test results? To address this issue, correlations between scores in Memrise and post-tests were examined in two different scenarios: a) when Memrise usage was obligatory (Unit 3), b) when usage of Memrise was voluntary (Unit 5). In both cases Kendall's tau was statistically significant (1-tailed), so it is legitimate to claim that high scores in Memrise coexist with high test results. However, interestingly, as far as voluntary usage is concerned, the correlation was decidedly higher and significant at a higher level (tau=0.5, $p < 0.001$, df=36 whereas in obligatory usage tau=0.34, $p < 0.01$, df=38). The results are shown in *Table 14* and *Table 15*. This may lead to the conclusion that there could be some unexamined, latent variable (probably a motivational one) that could have influenced the usage of the application for Unit 5.

*Table 14: Correlation between U3 Memrise score and U3 post- test*

| | |
|---|---|
| Kendall's tau | 0.34 |
| Sig. (1-tailed) | 0.001 |
| N | 40 |

*Table 15: Correlation between U5 Memrise score and U5 post-test*

| | |
|---|---|
| Kendall's tau | 0.500 |
| Sig. (1-tailed) | 0.000 |
| N | 38 |

As correlation results make the relation between Memrise usage (based on the number of Memrise points collected by the study participants, i.e. the Memrise score) and test results very probable, it was of interest to the author to check if there was a minimal level of Memrise score which needed to be gained to improve the overall test score (as the sample for Unit 5 was too small, this analysis could be performed only for Unit 3). To perform this analysis, a t-test for independent samples was used. The students were divided into two groups: below 50,000 points in Memrise U3 and above this score (see *Table 16*). The t value (-2.93) showed that the results in the Unit 3 post-test were significantly different (1-tailed $p < 0.01$). The t value in the t-test for groups with a lower minimum was not significant (e.g. for 48,000 points t= -1.25) while values for divisions with a higher minimum were still statistically significant (e.g. for division at a level of 60,000 t= -3.3, p<0.01). However, it should be taken into account that the minimum performance score in Memrise displayed by a statistical test is related to the sample magnitude, e.g. in the case of a minimum of 48,000 points, there were only 5 students in the "below minimum" group.

*Table 16: Results in U3 post-test for groups with/without minimum in Memrise U3*

| Group | N | U3 post-test Mean | t | p (one-tailed) |
|---|---|---|---|---|
| Below 50,000 in Memrise U3 | 7 | 26.07 | -2.934 | 0.003 |
| More than 50,000 in Memrise U3 | 33 | 40.85 | | |

A similar analysis was performed in search of a maximum Memrise score, where further learning did not improve the post-test results. The t-test showed that the level of 85,000 points could be considered as a cut-off point, beyond which more Memrise activity did not lead to better test results, as while the t-value (t=1.48) was significant, *t* for groups with a lower maximum was significant in the division based on a score of 85,700 points (t = -1.91 and p<0.05, one tailed). Again, the score pointing to over-learning is probably only an approximation, as the sample was quite small. The results are shown in *Table 17.*

*Table 17: Results in U3 post-test for groups with/without maximum in Memrise U3*

| Group | N | U3 post-test Mean | t | p (one-tailed) |
|---|---|---|---|---|
| Below 85,000 in Memrise U3 | 27 | 36.15 | -1.48 | 0.07 |
| More than 85,000 in Memrise U3 | 13 | 42.65 | | |

The above analysis showed some relation between Memrise usage and test results. To determine if self-paced Memrise-based homework enhanced the acquisition of course material the analysis of regression was performed. The results show that in the prediction of the Unit 5 post-test results both scores – in Memrise for Unit 5 and for Unit 3 – were important. What seems to be quite interesting is that the result of the end of term test was also one of the predictors, while Unit 5 pre-test results were not (see *Table 18*). The model has a very high $R^2$=0.86, so there is ample evidence to claim that these variables were very good predictors in the explanation of the results of the post-test, and – looking at the partial correlations – had the biggest contribution in the explanation of voluntary Memrise usage. Perhaps a central conclusion to be drawn is that the work with Memrise was the most important factor determining the students' success, or the lack of it. Also, the voluntary usage of Memrise was an expression of general motivation to learning English, which on the other hand, could be seen in the involvement in course activity in Unit 3 and the end of term test results. However, it should be taken into account that both standardized beta and partial correlation for Memrise U3 score were negative (while Kendall's tau for these variables was slightly positive, although not significant). The results are presented in *Table 18.*

*Table 18: Regression analysis of the U5 post-test results*

| | **standardized beta** | **t** | **p (2-tailed)** | **partial correlations** |
|---|---|---|---|---|
| Constant | - | .437 | 0.665 | |
| Memrise U3 | -0.392 | -4.25 | 0.000 | -0.62 |
| U3 task in the end of term test | 0.195 | 2.25 | 0.03 | 0.39 |
| U5 pre-test | 0.131 | 1.47 | 0.15 | 0.26 |
| Memrise U5 | 0.870 | 9.592 | 0.000 | 0.87 |

To see how the variables are related to each other, an additional analysis of correlation was made. It showed that Memrise scores in Unit 3 and Unit 5 correlated positively, but not on a significant level (tau=0.17), while Unit 3 task results in the end of term test correlated both with Memrise U3 and U5 scores (0.56, $p<0.001$ and tau=0.27, $p<0.05$, respectively). In my opinion, such an arrangement of correlations and beta justifies – at least to a degree – the above mentioned hypothesis about the impact of students' general motivation on various aspects of learning and its results. It could also be said that the Memrise Unit 5 score is a result of general motivation and active *here and now* variables not observed in the study (e.g. difficulty of other exams, personal situation etc.). Such results are in line with the students' declarations about the most important factors of success in learning a foreign language (see *Figure 14*).

*Figure 36: The prediction of the post-test results*

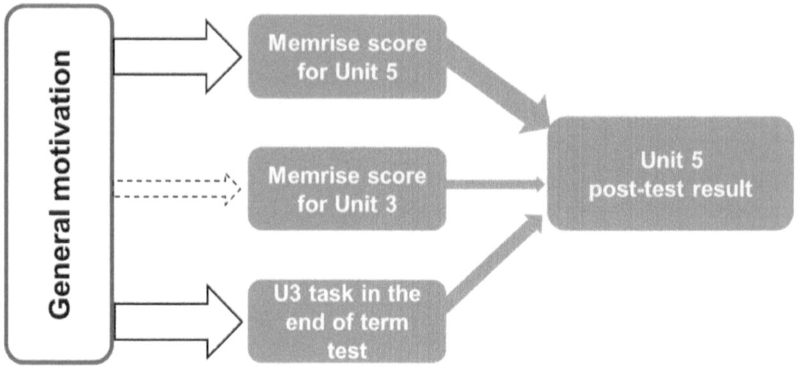


In other words, although results point to Memrise usage as a crucial factor determining success in the Unit 5 post-test, we might assume that it was only an expression of general attitude towards learning, which could be observed also in the end of term test results. However, as the result of the end of term test was not significant as a predictor of the Unit 5 post-test, motivation is not enough, and to achieve a good result students need to put at least minimal level of effort in (see the *Table 16* with minimum score in Memrise).

Consequently, we might assume that those students who had a relatively high Memrise score in Unit 5 and good results in U3 task in the end of term test would obtain the highest post-test scores in Unit 5. Other combinations of predictive variables could, but would not necessarily induce differences in post-test results. As the regression analysis showed, the impact of Memrise was more important, thus there should emerge a hierarchy of results:

- The above mentioned group should obtain the highest scores (high results in both Memrise U5 and U3 task in the end of term test).
- The second group should comprise students who had high results in Memrise U5 but poor results in the U3 task in the end of term test.
- The third group should be those who, despite low Unit 5 Memrise scores, gained a good result in the U3 task in the end of term test.
- Those students who obtained both low Memrise U5 scores and poor results in the U3 task in the end of term test would constitute the fourth group.

To check this reasoning, I divided the sample into four groups, depending on the scores in Memrise and the end of term test. The cut-off points were selected in such a way as to have similar numbers of members in every group and to ensure homogeneity within each group. The results confirmed the above presented reasoning: there was a hierarchy of the U5 post-test results. Moreover, the t-tests performed showed that the differences between Groups 1 and 2 were statistically significant ($t=4.79$, $p<0.001$). The differences between Groups 2 and 3, and between Groups 3 and 4 were not statistically significant. To conclude, having only a general motivation to learn, supported by actual effort leads to the best learning results (measured by the post-test).

*Table 19: U5 post-test results in sub-groups chosen on the basis of U5 Memrise score and Unit 3 task in the end of term test performance*

| Group No | N | U5 Memrise | U3 task in the end of term test | U5 post-test Mean | U5 Post-test SD |
|---|---|---|---|---|---|
| 1 | 10 | High | High | 41.8 | 18.18 |
| 2 | 9 | High | Low | 11.8 | 4.74 |
| 3 | 14 | Low | High | 10.7 | 5.91 |
| 4 | 5 | Low | Low | 9.0 | 10.15 |

To give a complete analytical description of the dependencies between variables, the author wished to calculate the regression of the post-test results in condition of obligatory Memrise usage. Unfortunately, due to an error in the system, the analysis was impossible as some important data was missing. Nevertheless, at this point it can be quite convincingly argued that:

- The learning process was effective.
- Memrise usage affected post-test results, and the impact of voluntary usage was probably higher than that of obligatory use (probably related to motivational interference).
- There was a minimum Memrise score that had to be achieved for post-test results to be improved.
- There is a cut-off score in Memrise, beyond which further practice is not very effective.

*Figure 37: Probable relation between voluntarily used Memrise and test scores (regression curve estimation)*

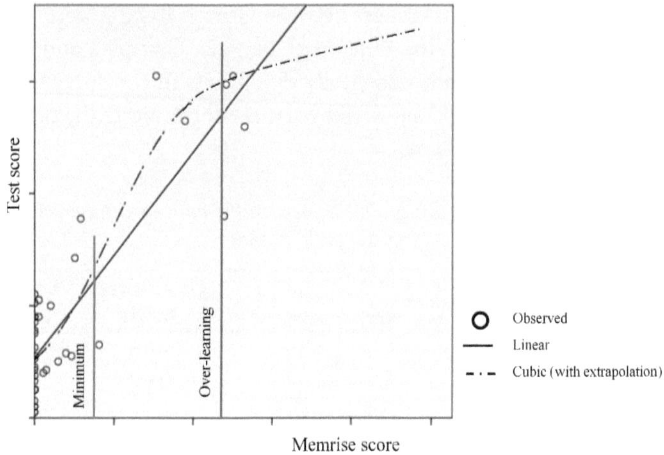


As signalled on the preceding pages, Memrise usage for Unit 5 was voluntary. It was then of fundamental interest to the author to establish what led participants of the study to use or abandon Memrise as an educational tool. Unfortunately, due to external restrictions imposed on the study, I was unable to merge data from the learning system with the questionnaire results. Therefore, such an analysis was performed separately. Firstly, a regression analysis was calculated to see if voluntary usage of Memrise for Unit 5 could be explained by other variables. The $R^2$=0.45 indicates that some of the volatility of U5 Memrise scores could be explained, but the only significant predictor was the U5 pre-test results. The contribution of other variables was not significant, at a level of 0.05, although the significance of the score in Memrise U3 was on a tendency level ($p<0.1$, the results are shown in *Table 20*).

*Table 20: Regression analysis of voluntary Memrise use*

| | Standardized beta | t | p |
|---|---|---|---|
| (Constant) | | -1.90 | 0.068 |
| U3 Memrise score | 0.323 | 1.90 | 0.066 |
| U5 pre-test results | 0.396 | 2.74 | 0.016 |
| U3 task in the end of term test | -0.236 | -1.08 | ns |
| end of term test | 0329 | 1.62 | ns |

These results suggest that the model is rather weak, and we could only say that the reason for voluntary Memrise usage was student motivation and English knowledge (which is probably an effect of earlier work caused by motivation). This leads to the conclusion that voluntary Memrise usage reflected a rather general attitude towards learning. To confirm this assumption a compilation of test results was created. A new variable, called the *test* was calculated as a mean result in three tests: U3 immediate post-test task, U3 task in the end of term test and the end of term test. These variables were put into the regression model. The result was in line with the previous reasoning: both variables, i.e. scores in Memrise U3 and new variables were significant predictors of the scores in voluntary Unit 5 Memrise usage (the results are presented in *Table 21*). However, the relatively low $R^2$ of the model ($R^2$=0.32) indicates that we still can explain only a part of the analyzed phenomenon.

*Table 21: Regression analysis of voluntary Memrise use*

| | **Standardized beta** | **t** | **p** |
|---|---|---|---|
| (Constant) | | -2.88 | 0.01 |
| U3 Memrise score | 0.359 | 2.45 | 0.02 |
| test | 0.321 | 2.19 | 0.04 |

On the other hand, it might have been the case that the application itself was not "captivating" enough for students to use it. If this was not true, the correlation between Memrise scores in U3 and U5 should be higher than correlations between Memrise scores and the *test* variable introduced above. As the correlation between Memrise scores was not significant (tau=0.17), while all other correlations were significant at $p<0.001$ (see *Table 22*), we could interpret the result as not contradicting the above reasoning. As the highest correlation was observed for the new variables (sum of Memrise scores in both voluntary and obligatory conditions), self-motivation was the main factor behind Memrise usage, and the application, though effective, could have been more "captivating".

*Table 22: Correlation between 'test' variable and Memrise scores*

| | **tau** | **P (one-tailed)** |
|---|---|---|
| U3 Memrise score | 0.29 | 0.004 |
| U5 Memrise score | 0.28 | 0.009 |
| Sum of Memrise scores | 0.41 | 0.000 |

As investigating the issue of Memrise's attractiveness to the study participants would be of relevance to teaching practice, the author again divided the students into four groups. This time the division criteria were: a) U3 Memrise score and b) U3 post-test results.

If the above assumption is correct, students who had high U3 Memrise scores and high U3 post-test results should also have the highest U5 Memrise scores. If the assumption is wrong, we should observe some changes, as those students who had low Memrise scores and low post-test results could have changed their attitude and decided to work more with Memrise.

The results (see *Table 23*) demonstrate beyond any doubt that there was a clear hierarchy of U5 Memrise scores. The mean in Group 1 was significantly higher than the mean in any other group (relatively: $t_{(1-2)}=2.14$, $p<0.05$; $t_{(1-3)}=2.84$, $p<0.05$; $t_{(1-4)}=2.89$, $p<0.01$). There was no large modification of student behaviour, and those who were good in Memrise Unit 3 remained good in Memrise Unit 5; on the other hand, those who were poor in Memrise Unit 3, stayed poor in Memrise Unit 5. Likewise, the correlation between U3 post-test results and the end of term test results remained concordant with the above reasoning (tau = 0.318, $p<0.01$, df=38).

*Table 23: Scores in U5 Memrise in sub-groups chosen on the basis of Memrise U3 score and post-test performance*

| Group | N | U3 Memrise | U3 post-test | U5 Memrise Mean | U5 Memrise SD |
|---|---|---|---|---|---|
| 1 | 10 | High | High | 75495 | 75273 |
| 2 | 11 | High | Low | 20355 | 40123 |
| 3 | 10 | Low | High | 6743 | 13327 |
| 4 | 9 | Low | Low | 2733 | 5498 |

To check if there was any difference between results in immediate post-tests after U3 and U5, the results were transformed onto a 0 to 1 scale (as a percentage of the maximum score). On such variables a paired t-test was calculated, which showed a marked difference between the results ($t=9.14$, $p<0.000001$). This means the average score in Unit 3 immediate post-test (0.63) was visibly better than in Unit 5 immediate post-test (0.26). As Memrise use was not the only difference (e.g. a slight difference in Unit content difficulty was a disturbance variable) we could not attribute the entire difference identified by the t-test result to Memrise alone. Nevertheless, as the achievement of the minimum score in Memrise (see *Table 16*) is one of the factors in test success, it makes it very plausible that the Memrise performance (or in other words: work/time invested in learning via the application) influenced post-test results in both cases.

The emerging picture shows that the usage of Memrise was related to some general factor – which could be composed of the attitude towards learning English, motivation, abilities, and attitudes towards m-learning. Unfortunately, due to the already mentioned restriction, it was impossible to merge all the necessary data; hence, in the further analysis only some aspects of student motivation and attitudes toward mobile learning are taken into account.

Before presenting these analyses, it should also be mentioned that according to the system data there were 21 students who obtained some points in Memrise for Unit 5. However, in Questionnaire 2, 22 students reported using Memrise. Although the difference was small, all the statistics presented should be treated with caution, because in such small groups, even one person can sometimes make a difference. Unfortunately, due to an error in the system, it was impossible to assign a Memrise score to a particular study participant.

There is a significant difference between Memrise Unit 5 Users and Non-Users in the amount of time devoted to study: 25% of those who claimed they did not use Memrise for Unit 5 (i.e. Non-Users) spent more than 2 hours per week learning, while among Memrise Unit 5 Users there was no such person, and heavy users spent only 1 to 2 hours learning (the percentage of students who spent less time learning with Memrise was not significantly different in both groups, see *Figure 38*).

From a different angle, this suggests that 25% of the students who spent a lot of time with Memrise in Unit 3 (obligatory practice) decided not to use it in Unit 5. Yet, although this number might seem large, these were actually three students who despite heavy Memrise Usage in Unit 3 decided to opt out of the Memrise course in Unit 5. In hindsight, an in-depth interview with these students would have provided valuable insight into the drop-out/opt-out factor.

*Figure 38: Time spent learning via Memrise*

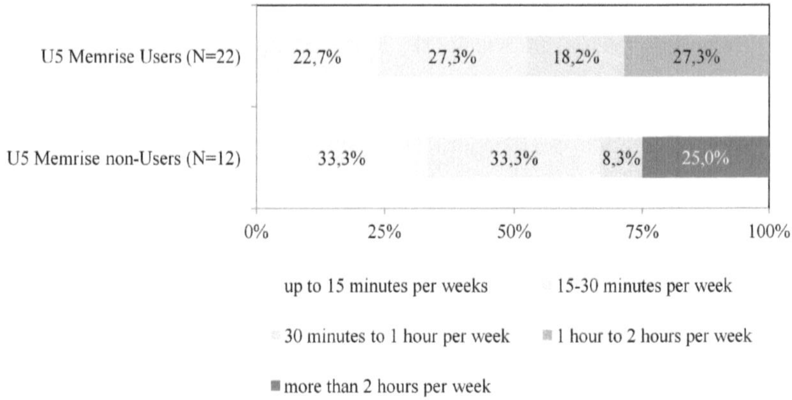


### *5.5.2.2 Concluding Remarks*

Having examined the test and Memrise performance related data, it could be claimed that only having a general motivation to learn, supported by actual effort (sufficient Memrise score) leads to the best learning results (measured by the post-test). It seems that the application was not "captivating" enough for some of the study participants to sign up for Unit 5 self-paced Memrise-based homework. This premise propelled Research Question 3 and led on to investigating the design of a mobile application that would address the issue of learning English for Medical Purposes.

## 5.5.3 Research Question 3: How did learners evaluate the Memrise-rooted MALL as an EMP learning experience?

To provide an answer to Research Question 3, the following questions from Questionnaire 2 were analyzed: *Rank Memrise on a scale from 1 to 5. Briefly justify your choice. Which 3 features of Memrise do you consider most important? Grade the following statements: Memrise helped me organize my learning better. / Memrise made the learning experience more personal. / Memrise was more convenient to use on a smartphone than on a desktop computer or a laptop/netbook. / Memrise was more convenient to use on a smartphone than on a tablet. / I found it convenient that I could use Memrise anywhere at any time. / A smartphone is a convenient tool for learning English for Medical Purposes. / I would be willing to upgrade Memrise to a paid version. / I would recommend Memrise as an educational tool to other medical students. / I found this way of learning motivating. / I will use Memrise in the future. / Compared with traditional paper-based homwe-work, the Memrise exercises were more interesting. / Thanks to Memrise I learnt more than I would in a traditional way.*

In Questionnaire 2, the participants were asked to rank Memrise on a scale from 1 to 5, where 1 was the lowest score and 5 was the highest score. As can be seen in *Figure 39*, half of Memrise Unit 5 Users awarded 4 points and the other half awarded 5 points, so the overall grade was 4.5. In the Memrise Unit 5 Non-Users group, 21% of the students awarded 3 points to Memrise, 50% awarded 4 points, 29% awarded 5 points and the overall grade was 4.2. Meanwhile, the overall grade for Memrise according to users who downloaded the mobile application from Google Play Store (1 million downloads; ranked by 45,706 users; date of access: 18 July 2015) is 4.6, with 32,956 (approx. 72%) users awarding 5 points, 8,400 (approx. 18%) users awarding 4 points, 2,173 (approx. 5%) users awarding 3 points, 896 (approx. 2%) users awarding 2 points and 1,281 (approx. 3%) awarding 1 point. None of the study participants, even among Memrise Unit 5 Non-Users, awarded less than 3 points. Therefore, even Memrise Unit 5 Non-Users were somewhat satisfied with the application and the reason for not using Memrise for Unit 5 did not lie only in Memrise itself. This claim is partially supported by the reasons the Memrise Unit 5 Non-Users provided for not attending the Memrise Unit 5 course, i.e. lack of time (8 responses), no internet access (1 response), having forgotten to do so (1 response), other duties and other university classes to pass (3 responses), low motivation (1 response).

*Figure 39: Memrise overall grade*

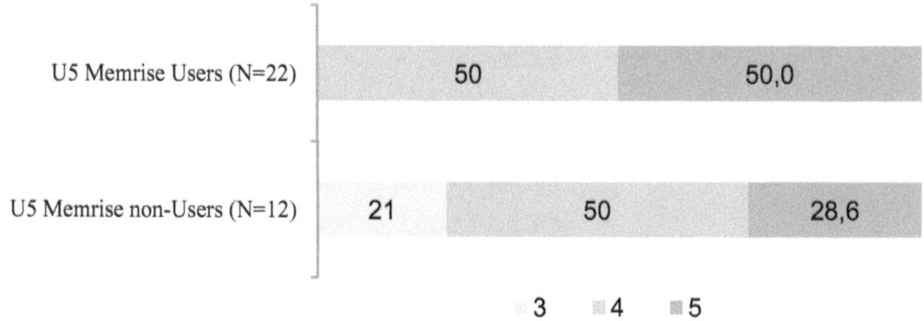


As far as Memrise's features as a mobile application are concerned (see *Figure 40*), its low price or being free of charge seemed to be important both to Memrise Unit 5 Users and Memrise Unit 5 Non-Users (82% vs. 86%, respectively). Not surprisingly, continuity of the learning process and cross platform use were more important to those students who actually used Memrise for Unit 5 rather than to those who did not (45% vs. 21% and 41% vs. 21%, respectively).The availability of audio files with pronunciation and intuitiveness/simplicity of use were equally important to 36% and 29% of Memrise Unit 5 Users and Memrise Unit 5 Non-Users, respectively. 27% of Memrise Unit 5 Users considered the possibility to add content important. Personalization of the learning process was slightly more important to Memrise Unit 5 Users than to Memrise Unit 5 Non-Users (22% vs. 21%, respectively). Interestingly, offline use was more important to Memrise Unit 5 Non-Users than to Memrise Unit 5 Users (50% vs. 23%, respectively), which might suggest that internet access, or the lack of it, e.g. when commuting, might be a factor encouraging or discouraging from using Memrise, even despite the offline mode. The ability to adapt the course to user needs was more important to Memrise Unit 5 Users then to Memrise Unit 5 Non-Users (18% vs. 7%, respectively). However, it should be mentioned at this point that the mobile version of Memrise lacks some of the functions available on desktop computers, laptops or tablets, e.g. it is impossible to eliminate the words the user considers unimportant or well-known from the pool of items to be studied. This issue was raised by a number of Memrise users who complained that they had to go through the words they knew and were unable to take them off the study list. This drawback might have affected the overall grade.

*Figure 40: The three most important features of MEMRISE*

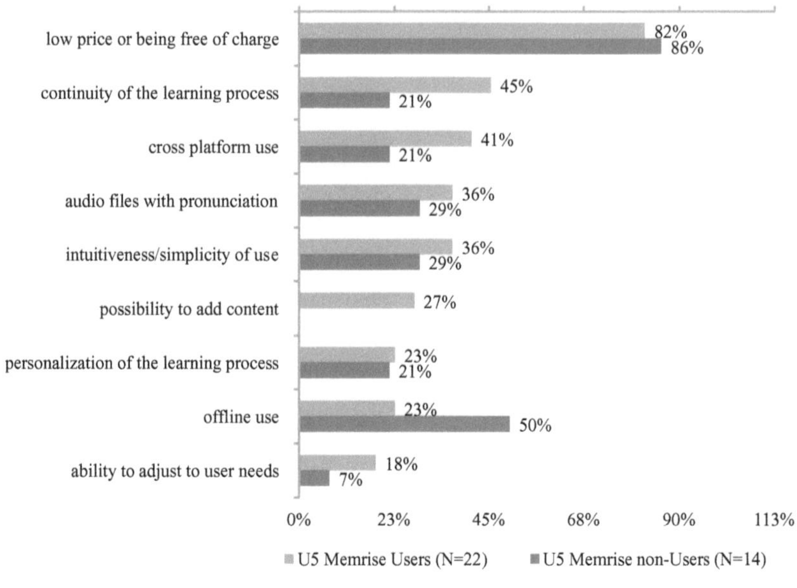

In Questionnaire 2, the study participants also ranked a number of Likert scale statements concerning the Memrise learning experience. The results are shown in *Figure 41*.

Generally speaking, it might seem surprising that the grade given by Memrise Unit 5 Non-Users was often higher than that given by Memrise Unit 5 Users, e.g. *Memrise helped improve my knowledge of EMP*- 4.7 and 4.4, respectively. Compared with traditional paper-based homework, the Memrise exercises were considered more interesting to Memrise Unit 5 Non-Users (4.5 and 4.4, respectively). More Memrise Unit 5 Non-Users would recommend Memrise to other medical students (4.5 and 4.3, respectively) and more Memrise Unit 5 Non-Users declared the use of it in the future (4.4 and 4.2, respectively).

*Figure 41: Post-project opinions*

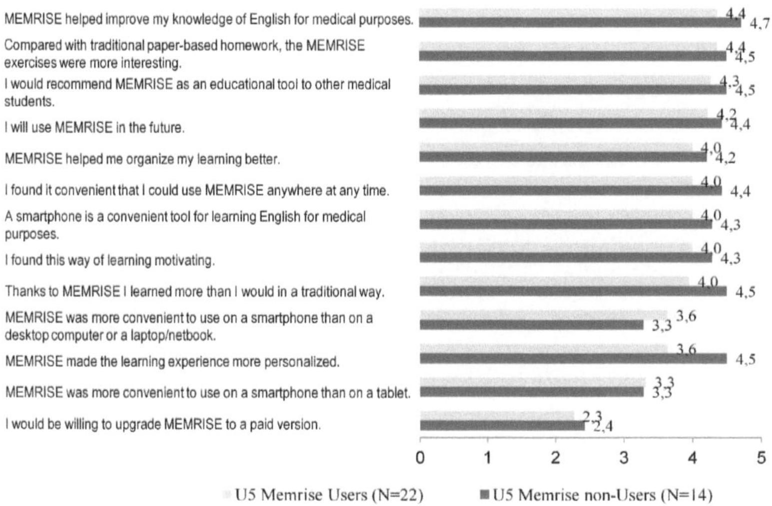


The Memrise experience from the obligatory Memrise Unit 3 course made the answers provided by Memrise Unit 5 Non-Users legitimate, however, the novelty factor might have played a more pronounced role in this case and the number of points awarded on the Likert scale might have been higher than that given by those study participants who took the Memrise Unit 5 course and had longer contact with the program, i.e. would be more knowledgeable about its drawbacks as well as advantages. Once again, Memrise Unit 5 Non-Users rated Memrise's convenience (*I found it convenient to use Memrise anywhere at any time*) slightly higher than Memrise Unit 5 Users (4.4 and. 4.0, respectively).

Although there appeared differences in assessing smartphones as a learning tool (4.3 for Memrise Unit 5 Non-Users and 4.0 for Memrise Unit 5 Users) and the rating of this way of learning as motivating (4.3 and 4.0, respectively) they were not statistically significant. Neither Non-Users nor Users would be willing to upgrade Memrise to a paid version (2.4 and. 2.2, respectively).

The differences between Memrise Unit 5 Non-Users and Memrise Unit 5 Users were greater in the case of *Thanks to Memrise I learnt more than I would in a traditional way* (4.5 vs. 4.0, respectively) and *Memrise made the learning experience more personal* (4.5 vs. 3.6, respectively), and were verging on statistical significance, nevertheless we can only talk of a tendency (p=0.55) rather than statistical significance.

As far as the efficiency of m-learning is concerned, in Questionnaire 1, 49% of the study participants considered m-learning efficient, 11% of the study participants strongly agreed with the statement, 8% percent of the participants disagreed with it, no one strongly disagreed but interestingly, 33% of the study participants did not have a clear view on the matter. The overall grade for m-learning convenience and efficiency was 3.6, whereas in Questionnaire 2 it increased to 4.0 and 4.5 for Memrise Unit 5 Users and Memrise Unit 5 Non-Users, respectively.

As far as the importance of the personalization of the learning process in concerned, in Questionnaire 1, 3% of the study participants strongly supported that view, 59% of the study participants were quite convinced that mobile learning makes the learning process more personal, 31% of the study participants did not have a clear view on the matter, 8% of the study participants disagreed with it and none of the study participants strongly disagreed with it. The overall grade for that factor was 3.6. In Questionnaire 2, the overall grade for that factor was 3.6 for Memrise Unit 5 Users and 4.5 for Memrise Unit 5 Non-Users. It might have been the case that some of the study participants who voiced dissatisfaction with the inability to take well-known vocabulary items off the Memrise vocabulary list in the mobile version of the program valued personalization to a greater extent, hence their higher notes in the question on personalization, but also lower rate of Memrise usage.

At one point, Memrise Unit 5 Users ranked Memrise slightly higher than Memrise Unit 5 Non-Users – they reported that the smartphone/mobile version of Memrise was easier to use than the regular desktop/laptop version (3.6 vs. 3.3, respectively). When the participants were asked whether they consider smartphones a convenient tool, the rate was 4.0 for Memrise Unit 5 Users and 4.3 for Memrise Unit 5 Non-Users.

In Questionnaire 1, 51% of the study participants stated that they preferred mobile devices to a desktop computer, 18% of the study participants stated the contrary and nearly 31% of the study participants were undecided. Also, at baseline, 64% of participants thought that smartphones are a convenient tool for learning English for Medical Purposes. That number increased to 77% in Questionnaire 2 and the number of the undecided decreased by nearly 8% (see *Figure 42*). One student (3%) strongly disagreed with the statement both in Questionnaire 1 and Questionnaire 2, nevertheless, the number of participants who disagreed with the statement dropped to zero. The overall grade for that question in Questionnaire 1 was 3.71, whereas in Questionnaire 2 it was 4.0 for Memrise Unit 5 Users and 4.3 for Memrise Unit 5 Non-Users. Thus, it might be concluded that the number of students perceiving a smartphone as a useful educational tool increased after their educational experience with Memrise and the smartphone itself as an educational tool was not the reason for opting out from the course.

*Figure 42: A smartphone is a convenient tool for learning English for Medical Purposes*

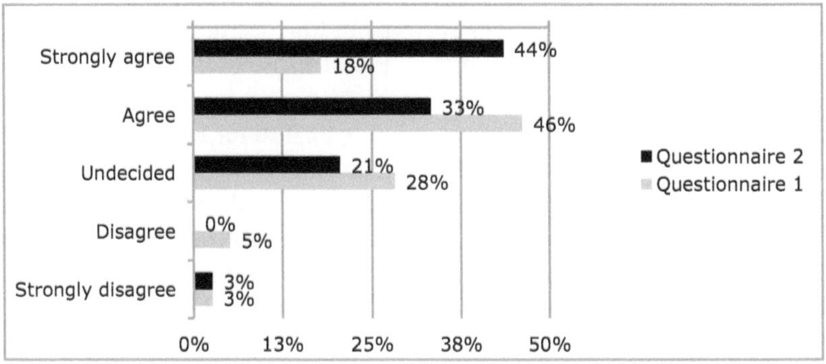


## 5.5.4 Limitations of the Study

The current study has limitations that should be acknowledged. As the study focused on a specific instructional context, i.e. first-year medical students learning English for Medical Purposes, the findings are not generalizable to other contexts. However, as this book deals with learning English for Specific Purposes, generalizations to other contexts need not necessarily be made. Moreover, the small number of participants and brief experimental period are a major limitation. The scope of the research project had to be adjusted to external restrictions imposed on the study by the medical university, to which the author is nonetheless grateful for the opportunity to conduct the study.

The author had to take into account the missing data resulting from, e.g. the lack of answers provided, the lack of some of the test scores or in one case inability to assign the Memrise score to a particular study participant. Hopefully, in each case the author exercised due diligence to maintain academic and analytical standards.

### 5.5.5 Concluding Remarks

The data from student responses before and after the research project demonstrate that the number of study participants who after the educational experience with Memrise considered smartphones to be a convenient tool for learning English for Medical Purposes increased by 13% and the number of the study participants who did not have a clear view on the matter decreased by 8%. The overall grade for m-learning convenience and efficiency increased from 3.6 initially to 4.0 and 4.5 for Memrise Unit 5 Users and Memrise Unit 5 Non-Users, respectively.

Memrise Unit 5 Users were less generous when grading Memrise features, probably due to the fact that they spent more time learning via Memrise and were more exposed to its shortcomings. The Memrise drop-out/opt-out factor might have been influenced by the co-occurrence of crucial medical exams, drawing student attention away from learning English for Medical Purposes to studying subjects with medical content. A number of Memrise Unit 5 Non-Users voiced the opinion that Memrise helped them organize their learning better, but it might be the case that those students, who despite impending medical exams found time to do the Memrise course, were better organised anyway, and Memrise usage did not have such a big impact on their learning habits.

Moreover, the results of the study clearly demonstrated that the study participants see themselves as agents of their language learning behavior. They consider learning as a proactive process and attribute success or failure rather to self-motivation than to the teacher.

To conclude, although the smartphone itself as an educational tool was not the reason for opting out of the Memrise course, the application itself was not "captivating" enough to change the learning habits of learners. It was then of interest to the author which Memrise features gained the greatest approval and disapproval of the study participants, and what they would expect from applications supporting the learning of English for Medical Purposes. For that purpose, the study participants were asked to answer a number of open questions, the answers to which will be discussed in the following chapter in the context of designing a mobile application that would best suit the needs of medical students.

# Chapter Six: Pedagogical Implications

## 6.1 Introduction

This chapter explores the issues concerning the design of a mobile application supporting the learning of English for Medical Purposes by medical students, i.e. a novel educational solution that emerged from the general discussion in the preceding chapters and insights from the study. The chapter first examines student comments regarding Memrise usage. Then general principles of mobile tasks are discussed. The chapter concludes with a description of the Mobile Medical English Companion.

## 6.2 Student Comments Analysis

The results of the statistical analysis of research data were discussed in detail in Chapter 5. However, as regards the development and integration of mobile learning environments, it is important to recognise the value of not only easily classified statistical data but also of the opinions of end users, learners. This section discusses learner contributions obtained in the open questions section of the post-project survey.

The study participants evaluated Memrise on a scale from 1 to 5 (see the discussion in Chapter 5). They were also asked to comment on the grade awarded to Memrise in the open questions section (63% of the study participants justified the grade awarded to Memrise). The study participants were also asked to comment on what they liked, did not like and would like to improve about Memrise.

The study participants voiced the following drawbacks of Memrise, which can be classified into: repetitiveness of items, time consuming process of learning, inconvenient answer entry mode (i.e. "speller"), lack of contextualisation, lack of an "ignore" mode in the mobile version of the program to omit well-known items, the fact that the mobile app is not supported by all types of mobile devices, problems with the offline mode, the mobile app being worse than the desktop version, revision issues and other (see *Figure 43*).

*Figure 43: Classification of student comments*

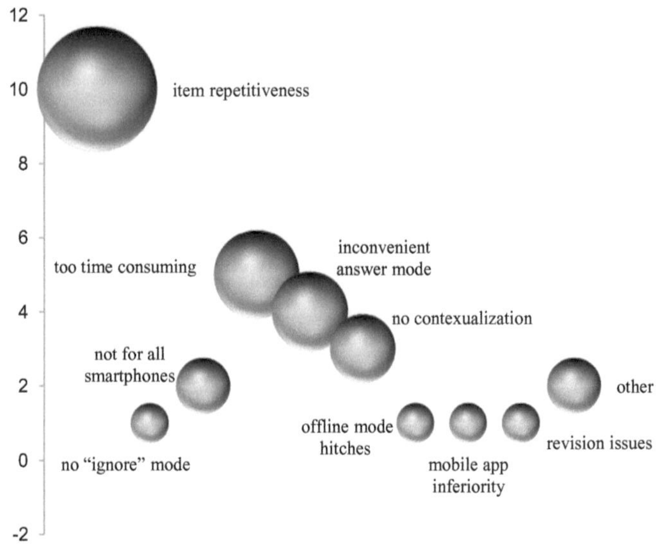


Those study participants who saw the need to improve the software (as some of the study participants said nothing had to be improved or admitted to not having thought about possible improvements) suggested a number of improvements discussed below:

- *The availability of a database of words and their translations with pronunciation* – Memrise software solutions enable course learners/users to preview a list of items for a given learning level (with the "opt out" option), however, only in the desktop version of the program; and the complete course database is available only to the course creator.
- *Exercises involving the use of items in context/Presentation of items in sentences* – Although Memrise allows learning strings of words, the types of exercises available on Memrise do not support context-sensitive ways of vocabulary learning (i.e. otherwise that providing a word in a sentence/context in the "definition" or "comments" box). Similarly, the postulated introduction of *translation of whole sentences* – although technically possible, at the moment, would be utterly inconvenient and inefficient due to software limitations.
- *Allowing alternate answers* – The only alternate answers allowed by Memrise are those pre-defined by the course creator.

- *Multiple-choice questions* – Although Memrise enables multiple choice answers, the question format does not allow typical multiple choice solutions, e.g. content related Question-Answer items. It is rather a translation matching exercise that fails to make the most of the multiple choice question potential.
- *Division into thematic sections with varying levels of difficulty* – The two courses offered to the study participants were divided into thematic sections devised in cooperation with the course teacher, but which did not encompass varying levels of difficulty, due to the fact that after university internal placement tests the study participants were to be a homogenous B2 CEFR group. Nevertheless, this point will be raised further in this chapter with relation to possible ways of constructing learning modules.
- *More/Fewer spelling exercises*– The usefulness of spelling exercises remains a contentious issue. Some of the study participants voiced the need to practice spelling (or typing in whole phrases, as mentioned above), whereas others pointed to spelling exercises as very inconvenient as regards the answer mode (and leading to item repetitiveness in the case of an obvious typo).

Some comments suggesting, e.g. *improved course search/tagging* or *greater availability of courses targeted at medical students* referred to general features of Memrise and were not related to course design itself.

Overall, student opinions provided insight into how to move beyond teaching vocabulary equivalents, so that the novel education model would encourage the students to use mobile technologies in learning English for Medical Purposes to achieve to their potential within a limited time framework.

## 6.3 New Educational Framework

21st century learners often request content accessible from the latest handheld devices. Herrington and Herrington (2007) discuss the shift in understanding learning; a shift caused, among others, by technological developments. Among the dimensions of learning affected by these developments, along with technology tools, Herrington and Herrington enumerate, for example, course design, time and place, knowledge base, resources, support, mode or professional learning, i.e. ESP learning context. All this calls for developing a new theoretical framework for learning and teaching English for Medical Purposes.

Over recent decades, course design has become more open-ended and flexible, with time and place distributed in such a way so as to best suit the contexts of the learners. Learning has also become more collaborative, networked and community based, which is clearly demonstrated by attitudes to knowledge. Knowledge is now perceived as a community-built construct, rather than something encyclopaedia-based. Also, transfer of knowledge is significantly simpler and it is becoming easier and easier to become more knowledgeable if needed. Professional learning less frequently takes place in the context of fixed time and date "one-size-fit-all" courses and group events, but more and more often the focus is placed on personal development and personalised learning.

> "The challenge for the educators and technology developers of the future will be to find a way to ensure that this new learning is highly situated, personal, collaborative and long term; in other words, truly learner-centred learning."
>
> (Naismith et al. 2004: 36, in Herrington – Herrington 2007)

Yet, innovative technology-enhanced educational scenarios need to comply with the general principle that "pedagogy and learning theory are the driving forces rather than mobile technologies" (Milrad 2006: 30). Therefore, I postulate the development of a Mobile Medical English Companion (MMEC) as an educational solution designed to support the learning of English for Medical Purposes to students at the Medical University.

Despite the existence of "all purpose" vocabulary trainers, creating both an appealing and effective medical vocabulary trainer is still a challenge. Although the study participants were obliged to complete an English for Medical Purposes course, they pointed to self-motivation as the key factor of successful learning. Following Coon and Mitterer (2007: 408) for intrinsically motivated learners "a certain amount of challenge, surprise, and complexity makes a task rewarding", whereas extrinsically motivated learners wish "to take the fastest, most direct route to a goal, not the most creative". Perhaps a well-designed mobile application would develop intrinsic motivation even if learners reach for it for extrinsic reasons, i.e. to decrease learning time.

The Mobile Medical English Companion would support language performance, as, to the author, performance support lies at the core of the unique pedagogic advantages m-learning offers in this field. A Mobile Medical English Companion can add value to the classroom teacher-led training system in the areas of vocabulary learning and review, quick reference, quizzes or games. The aim of developing the Mobile Medical English Companion is to encourage and develop new pedagogically sound learning strategies among university students who are already quite competent with u-technologies.

It is important to design and develop learning modules that will be effective in a mobile format, as the content for mobile devices needs to be created with mobile devices in mind. To reiterate, this should not be CALL content published in such a way so as to be readable on mobile devices, but custom designed mobile language learning solutions with a focus on performance support.

On a technical note, the creation of the Mobile Medical English Companion involves creating a "central repository" of materials as well as appropriate software compliant with will Android, Blackberry, Windows Phone or iPhone to accommodate the most popular operating systems. Responsive course design (RCD) tools need to be implemented to accommodate for various desktop sizes and different device types (as the medical university does not provide learning devices, it is BYOD – bring your own device, and in this particular case BYOP – bring your own phone, learning). Also the application design needs to overcome a set of limitations of m-learning, such as, for example, small screen environments (this developmental hurdle can be overcome, e.g. by scrolling options).

Attention needs to be paid to the appropriate theoretical underpinnings as well as pedagogical assumptions of the Mobile Medical English Companion. The importance of time-efficient training is greater now than ever, and essential in the case of medical students, as English for Medical Purposes instruction lasts for 2 years only. Following Kukulska-Hulme (2000), for the purpose of globalised work environments, learners "need to build up repertoires of words and structures that will allow them to use their knowledge in an active way" over four semesters of learning. It is crucial that medical students benefit from both traditional classroom instruction, as well as the digital format of learning by means of enhanced and redesigned educational processes, preferably with the aid of the Mobile Medical English Companion providing the scaffolding for in-class language performance.

Mobile assisted language learning is often accused of being "one step forward for the technology, two steps back for the pedagogy" (Mioduser et al. 1999: 758). Online vocabulary trainers have both affordances as well as limitations. Despite interesting and innovative design (e.g. the award-winning fiszkoteka.pl) existing mobile learning tools require sophistication to suit the needs of medical students. On a pedagogical note, as a mobile assisted language use solution, the Mobile Medical English Companion needs to cater for a shift from low mobility and low contextuality to high mobility and high contextuality concepts (*Figure 44*).

*Figure 44: A shift in the MALU paradigm*

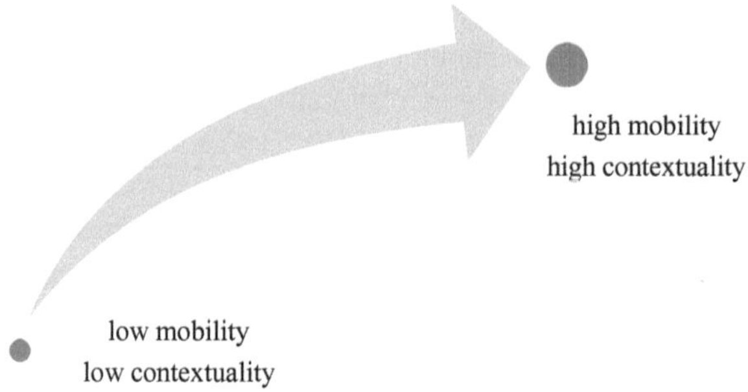


Also, it needs to involve bite-sized concise knowledge modules to sustain learner involvement, as well as comply with the informal "on the move" learning contexts. Following Milrad (2006: 29) innovative educational practice should take into account 1) context, 2) challenge and 3) scenario, activities and tools. As regards context and educational setting, the Mobile Medical English Companion supports informal English for Medical Purposes learning contexts, and would serve as a lynchpin for enhanced in-class performance. The challenge is to design a vocabulary trainer that would be appealing and effective at the same time.

*Table 24: The aspects of innovative educational practice (after Milrad 2006) with regards to MMEC*

| | **Mobile Medical English Companion** |
|---|---|
| **Context** (i.e. educational setting) | informal learning context (language support for in-class performance |
| **Challenge** | creating a compelling and effective vocabulary trainer |
| **Scenario, activities and tools** | SRS mobile application with appropriated activities |

The author investigated the habits of mobile users and their inherent expectations regarding mobile assisted language solutions to see how to make the most of the opportunities for vocabulary training.

## 6.4 App Design

In a paper from 2013, Stockwell and Hubbard outline ten general principles for the design and implementation of mobile applications and tasks using native mobile functionalities (*Table 25*). They review literature, e.g. works by Herrington et al. (2009a) or Elias (2011), Doughty and Long's (2003) Language

Teaching Methodological Principles for CALL or Chapelle's (2001) principles for evaluation of CALL tasks to identify three groups of issues of relevance to MALL design (*Figure 45*). They also highlight the importance of Elias's principles suitable for MALL solutions: equitable use, flexible use, tolerance of error and instructional climate. Following these principles, content in MALL solutions should be delivered "in the simplest possible format" and "packaged in small chunks". MALL solutions should also support "situated learning methods" and "push regular reminders, quizzes, and questions to students" (Elias 2011: 148, in Stockwell – Hubbard 2013).

*Figure 45: Key issues in MALL design (after Stockwell – Hubbard 2013)*

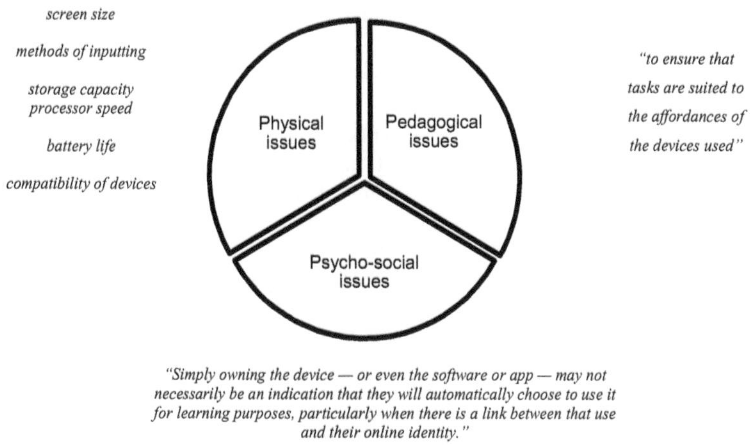


On a similar note, Herrington (2009: 134) offers guidelines for principles for mobile learning, of which real world relevance, providing sufficient time for exploration of mobile technologies, blended mobile and non-mobile learning, allowing spontaneous mobile learning and focus on non-traditional learning spaces seem to be crucial for the success of an application. Mobile solutions need to allow both knowledge construction, as well as language production.

*Table 25: Ten principles for the design and implementation of mobile applications and tasks using native mobile functionalities by Stockwell – Hubbard (2013: 8–10)*

| | |
|---|---|
| Principle 1 | Mobile activities, tasks, and apps should distinguish both 1) the affordances and limitations of the mobile device and 2) the affordances and limitations of the environment in which the device will be used in light of the learning target (Herrington *et al.*, 2009; Reinders & Hubbard, 2013). Crucially, if the fundamental goal is language learning, then these affordances and limitations should be directly connected in a principled way to second language learning research and theory (Chapelle, 2001; Doughty & Long, 2003). |
| Principle 2 | Limit multi-tasking and environmental distractions. Mobile environments, such as when commuting, by their nature are likely to be distracting, and multi-tasking is a natural part of that environment. We have increasing data that most people, including so-called digital natives, are not good at multi-tasking (Ophir, Nass & Wagner, 2009) and that it raises stress levels, increases error rates, and lowers productivity. As a result, it interferes with both deliberate and incidental language learning in both educational and workplace settings. |
| Principle 3 | Push, but respect boundaries. Research has shown that the push mechanism has the potential to prompt learners to action (e.g., Stockwell, 2013), but at the same time, learners have ideas of when and how frequently they would like to receive these reminders (Kennedy & Levy, 2008). Assuming learners are constantly connected with their mobile devices, it is possible to send content, activities, or simply reminders to learners regularly. These messages have the potential to shift attention to the learning task. However, they can also interrupt other more or equally valid activities, particularly in the workplace. A recommendation is to allow the user some control over when these push events occur, and to plan them for particular times to allow the learner to plan to accommodate them. |
| Principle 4 | Strive to maintain equity (Elias, 2011; Herrington *et al.*, 2009). In a classroom or other formal language learning setting, important issues to be sensitive to include whether the learner has a mobile device, what device the learner has in terms of compatibility and functionality, how consistent device connectivity is, and what the expense is for using that device for the planned operation. Reasonably equivalent non-mobile alternatives should be available if an inequity is apparent. |
| Principle 5 | Acknowledge and plan for accommodating language learner differences. As with other types of technology implementations, mobile learning should take into account a range of learning styles (Chun, 2001; Heift, 2002) as well as differences in comfort levels for learning in a public vs. a private space. For mobile devices, access issues such as visual acuity and manual dexterity for smaller keypads and touchscreens are also prominent concerns. |
| Principle 6 | Be aware of language learners' existing uses and cultures of use (Thorne, 2003) for their devices. Studies have shown that students may perceive their mobile devices as being for personal and social use rather than as educational tools (Liu, 2013; Stockwell, 2010). Some mobile applications may require developing new skills, but the more consistent a task or app is with existing uses, the more readily learners will likely accept it. |

| | |
|---|---|
| Principle 7 | Keep mobile language learning activities and tasks short and succinct when possible. As a corollary, divide longer tasks or activities into smaller, coherent chunks. This point is standard advice from other mobile learning frameworks (Elias, 2011; Herrington et al., 2009). Interruptions, which will occur predictably in many mobile environments, should trigger as little backtracking as possible when students are returning to the task. |
| Principle 8 | Let the language learning task fit the technology and environment, and let the technology and environment fit the task. If the assumption is that learners will be using a mobile phone at short intervals during the day (e.g., "dead time" between classes or other activities) in settings where it may be difficult to incorporate sound, then tasks should be developed that fit that technology and environment and still allow effective learning. If the assumption is that learners will be engaged in a task that requires longer chunks of time (20–30 minutes) and necessitates reading substantial text or other visuals from the screen and typing in short responses to questions, then appropriate technology (larger smartphones or tablets) and a more contemplative environment (e.g., library, classroom, or students' homes) would be called for. As Kukulska-Hulme (2013) notes, the mobility of the learner as well as of the technology must be considered. |
| Principle 9 | Some, possibly most, learners will need guidance and training to effectively use mobile devices for language learning. Hubbard (2013) makes a case for learner training in other domains of CALL, and there is no reason to believe that mobile language learning will be exempt from these challenges. Most of the preceding principles incorporate elements that are controlled by learners — teachers and developers may acknowledge them, but ultimately the implementation is in the hands of the mobile user. Learners unaware of the negative impact of multitasking or the environment in which they are using mobile devices, for example, need to be informed and trained in making their use as efficient as possible. Although the devices may claim to be intuitive, using them for language learning is not. Similarly, the literature on collaborative learning supports the idea that training for collaboration may be beneficial (Hampel, 2009) |
| Principle 10 | Recognize and accommodate multiple stakeholders. In the language classroom setting, adequate preparation and motivational support for teachers as well as learners must be provided. In the workplace, the impact of the potential ubiquity of mobile learning on co-workers, supervisors, and productivity in general should be considered, especially as it relates to Principle 2 above. Within both educational and workplace environments, mobile language learning is just one type of mobile learning that is likely to be occurring. There is potential for positive carryover from one learning domain to another, but also conflict as the needs for content learning and language learning merge or clash. |

Based on this analysis, and data obtained in the study, it seems legitimate to claim that an application supporting learning English for Medical Purposes should be user-friendly, but at the same time driven by guidelines of good teaching practice. Key features of a Mobile Medical English Companion would need to be resultant from the technological and pedagogical design issues, with detailed features as listed in *Table 26*.

*Table 26: Design issues in Mobile Medical English Companion*

**Technological Design**

- flashcard software with learning and revision based on a spaced repetition algorithm;
- elements of gamification, e.g. leader board, system of badges;
- possibility of setting up daily goals as well as term/mid-term related goals (e.g. "By the end of term I will have learnt…") with the space repetition algorithm adjusted to the academic situation (i.e. semester deadlines);
- reminders in the "pull" rather than "push mode", allowing user control over learning events (after Stockwell – Hubbard 2013, Principle 3);
- self-assessment mode ("I know/I don't know"/"opt out") and revision algorithm sensitive to that information;
- selective choice of modules, without going through Units 1 to 14 (as is the number of Units in the coursebook);
- flashcard creator: converting images/photos into flashcards;
- audio/text-to-speech support;
- limited multi-tasking available (after Stockwell – Hubbard 2013, Principle 2), taking into account differences in comfort levels for learning, e.g. in a public vs. a private space (after Stockwell – Hubbard 2013, Principle 5), sensitivity to access issues such as visual acuity and manual dexterity (after Stockwell – Hubbard 2013, Principle 5)
- offline mode (see Stockwell – Hubbard 2013, Principle 4);
- enabling "the carryover of the technology practices from the personal/social domain to that of language education" (consistent with Stockwell – Hubbard 2013, Principle 6)
- user manual available (after Stockwell – Hubbard 2013, Principle 9)

**Pedagogical Design**

- based on second language learning research and theory (after Stockwell – Hubbard 2013, Principle 1);
- self-contained, "bite-sized" modules (after Stockwell – Hubbard 2013, Principle 7);
- data set divided in such a way so that levels of difficulty correspond to the course grading system;
- accounting for a range of learning styles (after Stockwell – Hubbard 2013, Principle 5);
- adjusting to learning styles (as in *intelligent tutoring system* suggested by Ghadirli and Rastgarpour 2012);
- taking into account changes of motivation over time/motivation flux;
- allowing the learning of formulaic language ("language chunks", "lexical bundles");
- allowing the language learning task fit the technology and environment (Stockwell – Hubbard 2013, Principle 8).

Clearly the technological and pedagogical issues remain intertwined, e.g. ideally the spaced repetition algorithm should take into account deadlines imposed on students through institutionalised learning (i.e. the date of end-of-term tests) as well as adjust the setting of personal learning goals to the academic situation (i.e. calculate the suggested number of items to be learned daily/weekly/monthly to complete the whole course in time based not only on the assumed time frame and number of items in the Unit but also based on the self-assessment mode/"opt out" mode).

The Mobile Medical English Companion should also enable selective learning, i.e. choice of modules, without a module-by-module progression through Units 1 to 14 (as this is the number of chapters in the coursebook). Selective and bite-sized learning would also be important in the case of informal learning contexts, where it is crucial to allow the tasks to fit both the technology and the environment.

One of the more difficult issues in MMEC would be to account for comfort levels for learning, e.g. in a public or a private space, as the author believes that these learning environments should be supported by different types of activities. Public spaces, such as accessing learning material while commuting, or in so-called "dead-time" require limited multi-tasking due to the number of distractions or inconveniences (e.g. noise or poor data streaming). Therefore, apart from a regular "audio off" option, MMEC should allow the user to function in two modes: "on the move" and "feel at ease". The choice of the appropriate mode would determine the types of exercises available. For example, the "on the move" mode would offer exercises that do not require too much manual dexterity, e.g. it would disable the "speller" exercise, requiring careful entering of characters so as not to cause an obvious typo that would have impact on the revision algorithm.

*Figure 46: Comfort level adjusted MMEC modes*

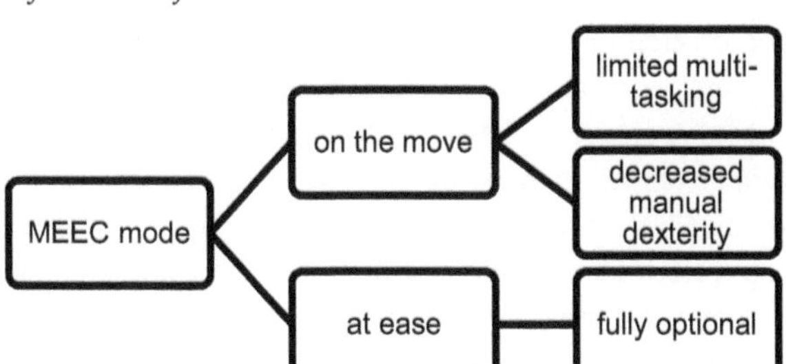

Another issue verging on the border of technological and pedagogical design is the question of reminders, and their control. As mentioned in Chapter 3, and as Stockwell and Hubbard emphasise in Principle 3, reminders inappropriately delivered to the application's end user in push mode may discourage the learner from using the software. On the other hand, they are one of the most frequently used methods to sustain motivation. A successful MMEC would need to account for changes to the motivation flux, i.e. changes of motivation over time, as well as the fact that, as mentioned above, in the case of institutionalised learning, motivation is often external. Allowing end users to exercise a considerable degree of control over the reminders makes the learning process even more personalised, and thus more likely to be successful. A key prerequisite is to provide "optimal levels of challenge, control, and interest" that facilitate the experience of *flow* (Dornyei 2005: 82). Introducing captivating tasks sustains "a particularly intense focus and involvement in an activity, to the extent that we may even lose self-consciousness and a track of time amidst our absorption. Thus, flow can be seen as a heightened level of motivated task engagement, leading to improved performance on a task; in many ways it is the optimal task experience" (Dornyei 2005: 82).

One solution to evoke and sustain motivation can be to introduce elements of gamification, such as a leader board, for example. Also, as MMEC is intended for a particular class-based context, application users might benefit from a system of badges, with avatars being awarded based on MMEC score, especially if it introduces a humorous element related to studying medicine.

Due to the amount of content-related terminology medical students need to learn (i.e. anatomy, medical equipment and devices or skin conditions, among others), a tool converting images or photos into flashcards would be an important feature of MMEC. Such solutions have already been adapted in some flashcard software (e.g. fiszkoteka.pl), however, in the case of English for Medical Purposes it is especially important that the learning materials are of high quality, and that they have been created or evaluated by experts. The creation of MMEC would thus involve, apart from creating a language database, the creation of a virtual repository of photos or images to illustrate learning. It is often the case that images of photos available online often are not of sufficient quality to serve as a basis for learning medicine, or their terms of use do not allow commercial use. Nowadays, there are many voices that mobile learning should promote collaboration and collaborative knowledge creation. However, in the case of Medical English, the quality (and correctness) of resources is of utmost importance, thus the mobile application does not necessarily have to encourage learner-designed materials.

The collaboration and gamification elements can be accomplished on a different level, i.e. the leader board, or during in-class cooperation.

Another important point in the case of medical English is the question of pronunciation. Thus, apart from audio files to accompany learning objects, a text-to-speech module would constitute a highly useful function of MMEC as the typical text-to-speech software solutions available online are far from satisfactory as far as medical English is concerned. MMEC's text-to-speech and integrated dictation exercises would make learning tasks (e.g. taking a patient's history) more authentic. Such a solution has been adapted in, e.g. *Duolingo* language learning software, however, the program does not support English for Medical Purposes. The creation of MMEC would involve text-to-speech solutions such as those available, for example, in *Quizlet*, but with an extended database.

Nowadays, much research is being conducted into intelligent tutoring systems (e.g. see the discussion in Ghadirli – Rastgarpour 2012) recognising personalised learning styles. As one of the features of successful learning solutions is that they comply with theories of learning, and language learning theory in particular, ideally, the MMEC would be an intelligent system adapting to a preferred learning style.

Last but not least, since the Mobile Medical English Companion is to support institutionalised learning, i.e. learning in the context where course objectives are clearly set out, the MMEC's software should also take into consideration formal course requirements. Apart from Unit-based modules, the application could also cater for levels of difficulty corresponding to the course grading system, i.e. learning items would be divided into "sufficient for a 3", "sufficient for a 4" and "sufficient for a 5" categories.

Developing software that will supplement the English for Medical Purposes curriculum rests not only on technical solutions, but also on providing good learning practice and high quality resources. As the study demonstrated, there is a necessity to develop a novel educational model supporting the learning of English for Medical Purposes with the use of handheld mobile devices because existing solutions are not fully responsive to the needs of medical students. The Mobile Medical English Companion is a learning solution aimed to encourage the learners to "perceive their mobile devices as appropriate vehicles for learning" (Stockwell – Hubbard 2013: 4).

*Figure 47: MMEC matrix components*

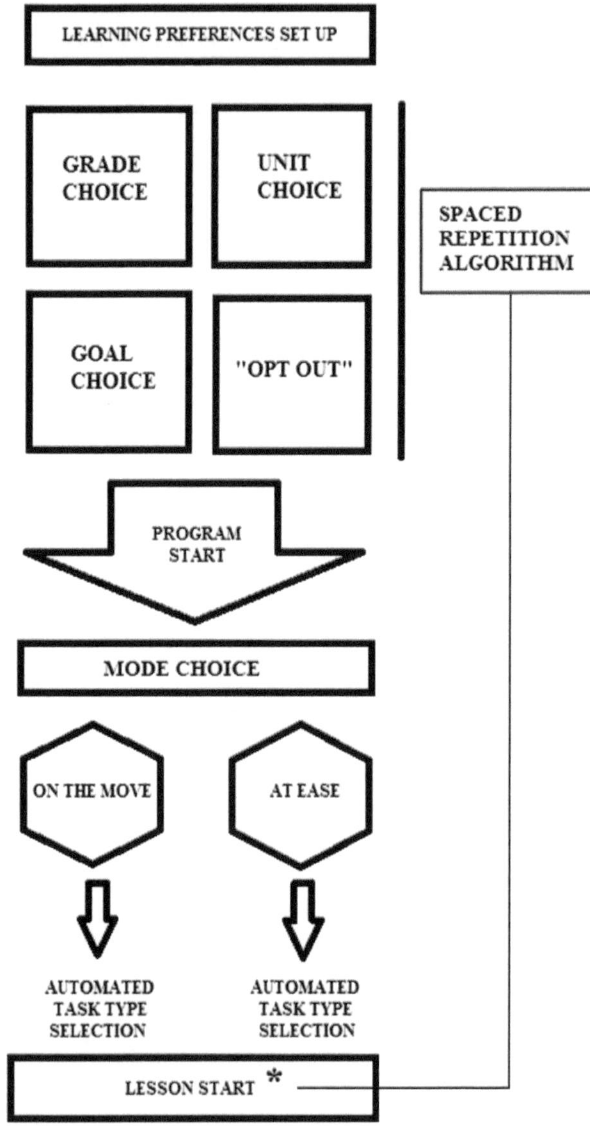


* active "opt out" function

## 6.5 Concluding Remarks

The main purpose of the final chapter was to present a novel educational model, the development of which was inspired and informed by the findings of the study. I have suggested developing a novel educational model to permeate pedagogy-informed use of mobile-assisted language learning solutions, as the gradually increasing access to reasonably priced portable technologies has led numerous language teachers to adopt mobile technologies into their everyday practice (Stockwell – Hubbard 2013, Oblinger – Oblinger 2005). Mobile-assisted learning solutions are an emerging discipline in the area of ESP education. It is important to collect research data on their use to optimise the mobile-assisted teaching of English for Medical Purposes. The ubiquitous nature of online language tutors points to their potential to become more than digital domain-specific word lists (see recent developments in Intelligent Tutor Systems or Mobile Human Computer Interaction) used in situations which require the assimilation of large amounts of information. Informed by the data obtained, it can be stated that this technology has the potential to, at worst, decrease test preparation time, and at best transform English for Specific Purposes practice. It is therefore important to capture the dynamic nature of the concept, to best assess which aspects of such a novel educational model supporting continuous and situated learning ought to be given prominence at the design and implementation stage.

Learning applications should emerge in the process of interaction between software developers, teachers and end users. The process of designing and implementing the Mobile Medical English Companion requires the availability of infrastructure and a number of advanced technological solutions. Appropriating the existing applications for the purpose of learning and teaching English for Medical Purposes is not sufficient and the situation calls for an innovative solution. However, the construction of the Mobile Medical English Companion will require a considerable amount of work, as well as a substantial amount of funding and cost investment, which are obviously barriers to implementing the model at short notice. Nonetheless, ongoing cooperation between the EMP teachers and mobile learning software developers is taking place, as a key prerequisite for the Mobile Medical English Companion to be successfully implemented.

Finally, it is important to reiterate that in the ongoing pursuit of innovative effective learning and teaching methods it is of utmost importance to find a "balance between the timeless and the up-to-date" (Turula 2015: 91). What the driving force for innovative technology-enhanced educational practices should be is research informed pedagogy, rather than mobile technologies themselves.

# References


Adams Smith D. (1984): "Medical discourse: Aspects of author's comment", *English for Specific Purposes* 3, 25–36.

Adolphs S. – Brown B. – Carter R. – Crawford C. – Sahota O. (2004): "Applying corpus linguistics in a health care context", *Journal of Applied Linguistics* 1(1), 9–28.

Åkerlind G. – Trevitt A. (1999): "Enhancing self-directed learning through educational technology: When students resist the change", *Innovations in Education and Teaching International* 36(2), 96–105.

Allegra M. – Fulantelli A. – Gentile M. – Taibi D. (eds.) (2008): *Emerging educational technologies and practices.* Palermo: Consiglio Nazionale delle Ricerche, Instituto per le Tecnologie Didattiche.

Alexander B. (2004): "Going nomadic: Mobile learning in higher education", *EDUCAUSE Review* 39(5), 28–35.

Allwright J. – Allwright R. (1977): "An approach to the teaching of medical English", in S. Holden (ed.), 58–62.

Anderson J. (1980): "The lexical difficulties of English medical discourse for Egyptian students", *English for Specific Purposes Newsletter* 37(4).

Andrews R. (2003): "Lrn Welsh by Txt Msg". Available at: http//news.bbc.co.uk/2/hi/uk_news/wales/279, 8701.stm (date of access: 27 November 2015).

Andrews R. – Haythornthwaite C. (eds.) (2007): *The Sage handbook of e-learning research.* London: Sage.

Anspach R. (1988): "Notes on the sociology of medical discourse: The language of case presentation", *Journal of Health and Social Behaviour* 29, 357–375.

Antić Z. (2010): "Analysis of student's errors in English for Medical Purposes", *Scientific Journal of the Faculty of Medicine in Niš* 27(3), 159–163.

Antić Z. (2014): "Medical studies in English: Shared learning", *Scientific Journal of the Faculty of Medicine in Niš* 31(2), 129–132.

Antić Z. – Todorović G.– Todorović L. (2013): "Writing biomedical research papers in English – a challenge for non-Anglophone authors", *Vojnosanit Pregl* 70(4), 424–428.

Arabski J. (ed.) (2002): *Z problematyki języków specjalistycznych.* Katowice: Wyższa Szkoła Zarządzania Marketingowego i Języków Obcych.

Arntz R. – Kühn B. (eds.) (2008): *Autonomes Fremdsprachenlernen in Hochschule und Erwachsenenbildung.* Bochum: AKS-Verlag.

Arrigo M. – Kukulska-Hulme A. – Arnedillo-Sánchez I. – Kismihok G. (2013): "Meta-analyses from a collaborative project in mobile lifelong learning", *British Educational Research Journal* 39(2), 222–247.

Aruba Networks Report (2014): "Are you ready for #GenMobile? How a new group is changing the way we work, live and communicate". Available at: http://www.arubanetworks.com/pdf/solutions/GenMobile_Report.pdf (date of access: 27.06.2015).

Atkinson D. (1992): "The evolution of medical research writing from 1735 to 1985: The case of the *Edinburgh Medical Journal*", *Applied Linguistics* 13: 337–374.

Atkinson J. (1957): "Motivational determinants of risk-taking behavior", *Psychological Review* 64, 359–372.

Attewell J. (2005): *Mobile technologies and learning: A technology update and m-learning project summary*. London: Learning and Skills Development Agency.

Attewell J. – Webster T. (2005): Engaging and supporting mobile learners. Mobile learning anytime everywhere: A book of papers from mLearn 2004. London: LSDA, 15–19.

Attewell J. – Da Bormida G. – Sharples M. – Savill-Smith C. (Eds.) (2003)

MLEARN (2003): Learning with mobile devices. London: Learning and Skills Development Agency. Available at: http://www.lsda.org.uk/files/pdf/1421.pdf (date of access: 20 November 2015).

Au S. (1988): "A critical appraisal of Gardner's social-psychological theory of second language learning", *Language Learning* 38, 75–100.

Ausubel D. (1968): *Educational psychology: A cognitive view.* New York: Holt, Rinehart & Winston.

Bailey K. (1986): *Class lecture*. Monterey: Monterey Institute of International Studies.

Baker F. (1992): *Item response theory: Parameter estimation techniques*. New York: Marcel Dekker.

Bakić-Mirić N. (2012): "Significance of creating a custom diagnostic English language test in English for Specific Purposes course at the University of Niš medical school", *Acta Medica Medianae* 51(1), 31–36.

Bandura A. – Schunk D. (1981): "Cultivating competence, self-efficacy, and intrinsic interest through proximal self-motivation", *Journal of Personality and Social Psychology* Vol. 41 No. 3, 586–598.

Barber C. (1962): "Some measurable characteristics of modern English scientific prose", *Gothenburg Studies in English* 14, 21–43.

Barber C. (1966): *Some measurable characteristics of modern scientific prose. Contributions to English syntax and phonology.* Stockholm: Alquist and Wiksell.

Bardovi-Harlig K. (2001): "Evaluating the empirical evidence: Grounds for instruction in pragmatics?", in K. Rose – G. Kasper (eds.), 13–32.

Barfield A. – Brown S. (eds.) (2007): Reconstructing autonomy in language education. Basingstoke: Palgrave Macmillan.

Basturkmen H. (2006): *Ideas and options in English for Specific Purposes.* Mawah New Jersey London: Lawrence Erlbaum Associates Publishers.

Basturkmen H. (2010): *Developing courses in English for Specific Purposes.* Basingstoke: Palgrave Macmillan.

Basturkmen H. – Elder C. (2004): "The practice of LSP", in A. Davies – C. Elder (eds.), 672–694.

Beetham H. – Sharpe R. (eds.) (2005): *Rethinking pedagogy for a digital age: Designing and delivering e-learning.* London: Routledge.

Belanger Y. (2005): Duke University iPod first year experience final evaluation report. Available at: https://cit.duke.edu/pdf/reports/ipod_initiative_04_05.pdf (date of access: 25 October 2015).

Belcher D. (2004): "Trends in teaching English for Specific Purposes", *Annual Review of Applied Linguistics* 24, 165–186.

Belcher D. (2006): "English for Specific Purposes: Teaching to perceived needs and imagined features in world of work, study, and everyday life", *TESOL QUARTERLY* Vol. 40, No. 1, 133–156.

Belcher D. (2009)a: "What ESP is and can be: An introduction", in Belcher D. (ed.), 1–20.

Belcher D. (2009)b: *English for Specific Purposes in Theory and Practice*. Ann Arbor: University of Michigan Press.

Belcher D. (2013): "The future of ESP research: Resources for access and choice", in B. Paltridge – S. Starfield, 535–551.

Belcher D. (ed.) (2009): *English for Specific Purposes in theory and practice.* Ann Arbor, MI: University of Michigan Press.

Belcher D. – Johns A.– Paltridge B. (eds.) (2011): *New directions in English for Specific Purposes.* Michigan: ELT.

Benfield J. – Feak C. (2006): "How authors can cope with the burden of English as an international language", *Chest* 129: 1728–1730.

Benfield J. – Howard K. (2000): "The language of science", *European Journal of Cardio-Thoracic Surgery* 18: 642–648.

Benson P. (2001): *Teaching and researching autonomy in language learning.* Harlow: Longman/Pearson Education.

Benson P. (2013) *Teaching and researching autonomy*. 2nd edition. Oxon, New York: Routledge Taylor and Francis.

Berge Z. – Muilenburg L. (eds.) (2013): *Handbook of mobile learning*. New York: Routledge.

Berliner D. – Calfee R. (1996): *Handbook of educational psychology*. New York: Macmillan.

Bhatia V. (1993): *Analysing genre: Language use in professional settings*. London: Longman.

Bhatia V. (2004): *Worlds of written discourse: A genre-based view*. London: Continuum.

Biber D. – Conrad S. (2004): "Corpus-based comparisons of registers", in C. Coffin – A. Hewings – O'Halloran K. (eds.), 40–56.

Biber D. – Connor U. – Upton T. (eds.)(2007): *Discourse on the move: Using corpus analysis to describe discourse structure*. Amsterdam: John Benjamins.

Biggs J. (1976): "Dimensions of study behaviour: Another look at ATI", *British Journal of Educational Psychology* 46, 68–80.

Biggs J. (1978): "Individual and group processes in study processes", *British Journal of Educational Psychology* 48, 266–279.

Biggs J. (1979): "Individual differences in study processes and the quality of learning outcomes", *Higher Education* 8, 381–394.

Bloor M. – Bloor T. (1986): *Language for specific purposes: Theory and practice*. Trinity College Dublin: Centre for Language and Communication Studies.

Boekaerts M. (2001): "Context sensitivity: Activated motivational beliefs, current concerns and emotional arousal", in S. Volet – S. Jarvela (eds.), 17–31.

Bosher S. – Smalkowski K. (2002): "From needs analysis to curriculum development: Designing a course in health-care communication for immigrant students in the USA", *English for Specific Purposes* 21, 59–79.

Bouhnik D. – Marcus T. (2005): "Interaction in distance-learning courses", *Journal of the American Society for Information Science and Technology* Vol. 57, Issue 3, 299–305.

Bow H. – Dattilo J. – Jonas A. – Lehmann C. (2013): "A crowdsourcing model for creating preclinical medical education study tools", *Acad Med.* 88(6): 766–770. Available at: doi: 10.1097/ACM.0b013e31828f86ef (date of access: 13 November 2015).

Breen R. – Lindsay R. (2002): "Different disciplines require different motivations for s/tudent success", *Research in Higher Education* 43(6), 693–725.

Brophy J. (1987): "Synthesis of research on strategies for motivating students to learn", *Educational Leadership* 45(2): 40–48.

Brown A. (ed.) (2006): Proceedings of Learning on the Move: Online Learning and Teaching Conference, Brisbane, Australia: Queensland University of Technology.

Brown D. (2000): *Principles of language learning and teaching. Fourth edition.* New York Pearson Longman.

Brown E. (ed.): (2001): Mobile learning explorations at the Stanford Learning Lab. *Speaking of Computers* 55.

Brown K. (2006): *Encyclopedia of Language and Linguistics 2nd edition.* Oxford: Elsevier.

Brunton M. (2009): "An account of ESP – with possible future directions", *English for Specific Purposes Issue* 3 (24), Volume 8. Available at: http://www.esp-world.info/Articles_24/An%20account%20of%20ESP.pdf (date of access: 7 April 2014).

Burden P. (1995): *Classroom management and discipline.* New York: Longman.

Burston J. (2013): "Mobile-assisted language learning: A selected annotated bibliography of implementation studies 1994–2012", *Language Learning and Technology* Vol. 17 No. 3, 157–225.

Buttner Zimmer A. (2007): *Activities, games, and assessment strategies for the world languages classroom.* New York, London: Routledge.

Byrd P. – Coxhead A. (2010): "On the other hand: Lexical bundles in academic writing and the teaching of EAP". University of Sydney papers in TESOL 5, 31–64. Available at: http://faculty.edfac.usyd.edu.au/projects/usp_in_tesol/pdf/volume05/Article02.pdf (date of access: 25 October 2015).

Canfield J. – Wells H. (1994): *100 ways to enhance self-concept in the classroom. 2nd ed.* Boston: Allyn & Bacon.

Carli A. – Ammon U. (eds.) (2007): *Linguistic inequality in scientific communication today. AILA Review* 20. Amsterdam: John Benjamins.

Carter-Thomas, S. – Rowley-Julivet E. (2008): "If-conditionals in medical discourse: From theory to disciplinary practice", *Journal of English for Academic Purposes* 7, 191–205.

Caudill J.G. (2007): "The growth of m-learning and the growth of mobile computing: Parallel developments", *International Review of Research in Open and Distance Learning* 2007, 8(2), 1–13.

Celce-Murcia M. (ed.) (2001): *Teaching English as a second or foreign language. 3rd edition.* Boston: Heinle & Heinle.

Chambers F. (1980): "A re-evaluation of needs analysis", *ESP Journal* 1(1), 25–33.

Chambers G.(1999): *Motivating Language Learners.* Clevedon: Multilingual Matters.

Chang C. – Sheu J. – Chen T. (2003: "Concept and design of ad hoc and mobile classrooms", *Journal of Computer Assisted Learning* 19(3), 336–346.

Chapelle C. (ed.) (2001): *Computer applications in second language acquisition: Foundations for teaching, testing and research*. Cambridge: Cambridge University Press.

Chapelle C. (2013): *The encyclopedia of applied linguistics*. New York: Wiley.

Charpy J. – Carnet D. (2014): "The European sTANDEM project for certification in medical English: Standards, acceptability and transgression(s)", *ILCEA* 19. Available at: http://ilcea.revues.org/2475 (date of access: 12 October 2014).

Chen C. (2010): "The implementation and evaluation of a mobile self- and peer-assessment system", *Computers & Education* 55, 229–236.

Chen C. – Chung C. (2008): "Personalized mobile English vocabulary learning system based on Item response theory and learning memory cycle", *Computers & Education* 51, 624–645.

Chen Q. – Ge G. (2007): "A corpus based lexical study on frequency and distribution of Coxhead's AWL word families in medical research articles", *English for Specific Purposes* 26: 502–514.

Cheng A. (2011): "ESP classroom-based research: Basic considerations and future research questions", in D. Belcher – A. Johns – B. Paltridge (eds.), 44–72.

Chinnery G. (2006): "Emerging technologies. Going to the MALL: mobile assisted language learning", *Language Learning & Technology* 10(1), 9–16.

Chun D. (2001): "L2 reading on the web: Strategies for accessing information in hypermedia", *Computer Assisted Language Learning* 14(5), 367–403.

Chung T. – Nation P. (2003): "Technical vocabulary in specialized texts", *Reading on Foreign Language* 15: 103–116.

Chung T. – Nation P. (2004): "Identifying technical vocabulary", *System* 32, 251–263.

Ciecierska J. – Jenike B. – Tudruj K. (2004): *English in medicine*. Warszawa: Wydawnictwo Lekarskie PZWL.

Clément R. (1986): "Second language proficiency and acculturation: An investigation of the effects of language status and individual characteristics:, *Journal of Language and Social Psychology* 5, 271–290.

Clément R – Dörnyei Z. – Noels A. (1994): "Motivation, self-confidence and group cohesion in the foreign language classroom", *Language Learning* 44(3), 417–448.

Cobcroft R. – Towers S. – Smith J. – Bruns A. (2006): Mobile learning in review: Opportunities and challenges for learners, teachers, and institutions. Proceedings of the Online Learning and Teaching Conference (OLT),

Brisbane: Queensland University of Technology. Available at: http://core.ac.uk/download/pdf/10876464.pdf (date of access: 25 October 2015).

Coffey B. (1984): "ESP – English for Specific Purposes", *Language Teaching* Vol. 17(1), 2–16.

Coffin C. – Hewings A. – O'Halloran K. (eds.) (2004): *Applying English grammar: Functional and corpus approaches*. London: Arnold.

Collins T. (2005): English class on the air: Mobile language learning with cell phones. The fifth IEEE international conference on advanced learning technologies (ICALT'05), 402–403.

Conole G. – de Laat M. – Dillon T. – Darby J. (2008): "Disruptive technologies, pedagogical innovation. What's new: Findings from an in-depth study of students' use and perception of technology", *Computers & Education* 50(2), 511–524.

Connor U. (2002): "New directions in contrastive rhetoric", *TESOL Quarterly* 36, 493–510.

Connor U. (2004): "Íntercultural rhetoric research: Beyond texts", *Journal of English for Academic Purposes* 3, 291–304.

Cook G. (2003): *Applied linguistics*. Oxford: Oxford University Press.

Cook V. – Singleton D. (2014): *Key topics in Second Language Acquisition*. Bristol: Multilingual Matters.

Coon D. – Mitterer J. (2007): *Introduction to psychology. Gateways to mind and behaviour. 11th edition*. Belmont: Thomson Wadsworth.

Cooney G. – Koegh K. (2007): "Use of mobile phones for language learning and assessment for learning. Paper presented at *MLearn 2007*." http://www.learnosity.com/files/learnosity-use-ofmobile-phones-for-language-learning-and-assessment-for-learning.pdf. (date of access: 10 July 2014).

Corbeil J. – Valdes-Corbeil M. (2007): "Are you ready for mobile learning?", *Educause Quarterly* 30(2), 51–60.

Corbeil R. – C. Pan – Sullivan M. – Butler J. (2007): "Enhancing e-learning through m-learning: Are you ready to go mobile?", in C. Crawford (ed.), 273–280.

Corder N. (2002): *Learning to teach adults. An introduction*. London and New York: Routledge.

Cornwell S. – Robinson P. (eds.) (2000): *Individual differences in foreign language learning: Effects of aptitude, intelligence, and motivation*. Tokyo: Japanese Association for Language Teaching.

Cortez P. – Roy D. (2012): "Screen interface design for mobile-assisted language learning in EFL context: A case study in Japan", *Journal of Language Teaching and Research* Vol. 3 No. 3, 353–368.

Covington M. (1998): *The will to learn: A guide for motivating young people.* New York: Cambridge University Press.

Coxhead A. (1998): *The development and evaluation of a new academic word list.* Unpublished MA thesis. University of Wellington, New Zeland.

Coxhead A. (2000): "A new Academic Word List" *TESOL QUARTERLY* Vol. 34 No. 2, 213–238.

Coxhead A. (2013) "Vocabulary in ESP", in B. Paltridge – S. Starfield, 115–132.

Coxhead A. – Nation P. (2001): "The specialised vocabulary of English for Academic Purposes", in J. Flowerdew – M. Peacock (eds.), 252–267.

Cranmer D. (1996): *Motivating high level learners.* Harlow: Longman.

Crawford C. (ed.) (2007): Proceedings of Society for Information Technology & Teacher Education (SITE) International Conference, Chesapeake, VA: AACE, 273–280.

Crawford Camiciottoli, B. (2007): *The language of business studies lectures.* Amsterdam: John Benjamins.

Crawford C. – Willis D. – Carlsen R. – Gibson I. – McFerrin K. – Price J. – Weber R. (eds.) (2006): Proceedings of Society for Information Technology & Teacher Education International Conference 2007, Chesapeake, VA: AACE.

Crookes G – Schmidt R. (1991): "Motivation: Reopening the research agenda", *Language Learning* 41, 469–512.

Csongor A. – Rébék-Nagy G. (2013): "Hedging in popular scientific articles on medicine", in *Acta Medica Marisiensis* 59(2), 97–99.

Cunningham D. – Hatoss A. (eds.) (2005): *An international perspective on language policies, practices and proficiencies.* Belgrave: FIPLV.

Dakowska M. (2005): *Teaching English as a foreign language. A guide for professionals.* Warszawa: Wydawnictwo Naukowe PWN SA.

Damon W. – Eisenberg N. (eds.) (1998): *Handbook of Child Psychology: Vol. 3. Social, emotional, and personality development. 5th ed.* New York: Wiley.

Davies A. (2001): "The logic of testing languages for specific purposes", *Language Testing* 18: 133–48.

Davies B. (2009): *Tools for teaching. 2 ed.* San Franciso: John Wiley & Sons.

Davies A. – Elder C. (eds.) (2004): *The handbook of applied linguistics.* Malden: Blackwell Publishing Ltd.

de Cássia Veiga Marriott, R. – P. Lupion Torres (eds.) (2009): *Handbook of research on e-learning methodologies for language acquisition*. Hershey: Information Science Reference.

Deci E. (1975): *Intrinsic motivation*. New York: Plenum.

Deci E. – Ryan R. (1985) *Intrinsic motivation and self-determination in human behavior*. New York: Plenum Press.

Demb A. – Erickson D. – Hawkins-Wilding S. (2004): "The laptop alternative: Student reactions and strategic implications", *Computers & Education* 43(4), 383–401. Available at: doi: 10.1016/j.compedu.2003.08.008 (date of access: 14 November 2015).

Demouy V. – Eardley A. – Kukulska-Hulme A. – Thomas R. (2010): "Using mobile devices for listening and speaking practice in languages: The L120 mobile project". Available at: http://oro.open.ac.uk/28605/ (date of access: 14 November 2014).

Demouy V. – Q. Kan – A. Eardley – Kukulska-Hulme A. (2013): "Using mobile devices for language learning in a higher education distance learning context: Motivations and behaviours". Available at: http://oro.open.ac.uk/38999/ (date of access: 14 November 2014).

Demouy V. – A. Kukulska-Hulme (2010): "On the spot: Using mobile devices for listening and speaking practice on a French language programme", *Open Learning: The Journal of Open and Distance Learning* 25(3), 217–232.

Dias J. (2002a): "Cell phone in the classroom: boon or bane?", *C@lling Japan* 10(2), 16–21.

Dias J. (2002b): "Cell phone in the classroom: boon or bane? Part 2", *C@lling Japan* 10(3) 8–13.

Díaz-Vera J. (ed.) (2012): *Left to my own devices: Learner autonomy and Mobile-Assisted Language Learning*. Language and Linguistics Special E-Book Collection, 2007–2012 Vol. 6. Bingley: Emerald Group Publishing Limited.

Doughty C. – Long M. (2003): "Optimal psycholinguistic environments for distance foreign language learning", *Language Learning & Technology* 7(3), 50–80.

Douglas D. (2000): *Assessing Languages for Specific Purposes*. Cambridge: Cambridge University Press.

Douglas D. (2013): "ESP and assessment", in B. Paltridge – S. Starfield (eds.), 367–383.

Dörnyei Z. (1994): "Motivation and motivating in the foreign language classroom", *Modern Language Journal* Vol. 78 No. 3, 273–284.

Dörnyei Z. (2001): *Motivational strategies in the language classroom*. Cambridge: Cambridge University Press.

Dörnyei Z. (2005): *The psychology of the language learner: Individual differences in second language acquisition*. Mahwah: Lawrence Erlbaum.

Dörnyei Z. (2009): *The psychology of second language acquisition*. Oxford: Oxford University Press.

Dörnyei Z. (ed.) (2003): *Attitudes, orientations, and motivations in language learning*. Oxford: Blackwell.

Dörnyei Z. – Csizér K. (1998): "Ten commandments for motivating language learners: Results of an empirical study", *Language Teaching Research* Vol. 2 No. 3, 203–229.

Dörnyei Z. – Kormos J. (2000): "The role of individual and social variables in oral task performance", *Language Teaching Research* 4, 275–300.

Dörnyei Z. – MacIntyre P. – Henry A. (eds.) (2014): *Motivational dynamics in language learning*. Bristol: Multilingual Matters.

Dörnyei Z. – Otto I. (1998): "Motivation in action: A process model of L2 motivation. *Working Papers in Applied Linguistics* 4, 43–69.

Dörnyei Z. – Schmidt R. (eds.) (2001): *Motivation and second language acquisition*. Honolulu: University of Hawaii Press.

Dubois B. (1980) "The use of slides in biomedical speeches", *ESP Journal* Vol. 1 No. 1, 45–50.

Dubois B. (1981): "The construction of noun phrases in biomedical journal articles", in J. Hoedt – R. Turner (eds.), 49–67.

Dubois B. (1983) "Paragraph structure of biomedical speeches: Preliminary report", in A. Manning – P. Martin – K. McCalla (eds.), 323–333.

Dubois B. (1985): "Poster sessions at biomedical meetings: Design and presentation", *English for Specific Purposes* 4, 37–48.

Dudley-Evans, T. – Bates M. (1976): *Nucleus: General science*. Harlow: Longman.

Dudley-Evans T. – St John M. (1998): *Developments in English for Specific Purposes: A multidisciplinary approach*. Cambridge: CUP.

Džuganová B. (2013): "English medical terminology – different ways of forming medical terms", *JAHR* Vol. 4 No. 7, 55–69.

Ebbinghaus H. (1885): Über das Gedächtnis: Untersuchungen zur experimentellen Psychologie. *New unchanged and unshortened edition*. Darmstadt: WBG.

Edwards P. (1974): "Teaching specialist English (with special reference to English for nurses and midwives in Nigeria)", *ELT Journal* 28, 247–252.

Eggly S. – Musial J. – Smulowitz J. (1999): "Research and discussion note the relationship between English language proficiency and success as a medical resident", *English for Specific Purposes 18(*2), 201–208.

Elias T. (2011): "Universal instructional design principles for mobile learning", *International Review of Research in Open and Distance Learning* 12(2), 143–156.

Ellis V. – Edwards A. – Smagorinsky P. (eds.) (2010): *Cultural-historical perspectives on teacher education and development. Learning teaching.* New York, London: Routledge Taylor & Francis Group.

Ewer J. – Hughes-Davies G. (1971): "Further notes on developing an English programme for students of science and technology", *English Language Teaching* 26(1,3).

Ewer J. – G. Latorre (1969): *A course in basic scientific English.* London: Longman.

Fallahkhair S. – Pemberton L. – Griffiths R. (2007): "Development of a cross-platform ubiquitous language learning service via mobile phone and interactive television", *Journal of Computer Assisted Learning* 23(4), 312–325.

Farrow R. – Arrigo M. – Kukulska-Hulme A. – Arnedillo-Sánchez I. (2010):

*Mobile Technologies in Lifelong Learning (MOTILL): Scientific Annotated Review Database.* MOTILL.

Ferguson G. (2001): "If you pop over there. A corpus-based study of conditionals in medical discourse", *English for Specific Purposes* 20, 61–82.

Ferguson G. (2013): "English for Medical Purposes", in B. Paltridge – S. Starfield (ed.), 243–262.

Ferris D. (2001): "Teaching writing for academic purposes" in J. Flowerdew – M. Peacock (eds.), 298–314.

Flowerdew L. (2013): "Needs analysis and curriculum development in ESP", in B. Paltridge – S. Starfield (eds.), 325–346.

Flowerdew J. – Peacock M. (eds.) (2001): *Research perspectives on English for Academic Purposes.* Cambridge: Cambridge University Press.

Gajek E. (ed.) (2015): Technologie mobilne w kształceniu językowym. Warszawa: Texter.

Gajewska E. – Sowa M. (2014): *LSO, FOS, Fachsprache…dydaktyka języków specjalistycznych.* Lublin: Werset.

Galloway D. – Rogers C. – Armstrong D. – Leo E. (1998): *Motivating the difficult to teach.* Harlow: Longman.

Galova D. (ed.) (2007): *Languages for Specific Purposes: Searching for common solutions.* Newcastle: CUP.

Gardner R. (1979): "Social psychological aspects of second language acquisition", in H. Giles – R. St. Clair (eds.), 193–220.

Gardner R. (1985): *Social psychology and second language learning: The role of attitudes and motivation*. London: Edward Arnold.

Gardner R. (2006) "The socio-educational model of second language acquisition: A research paradigm", *EUROSLA* Yearbook 6, 237–260.

Gardner R. – Lambert W. (1959): "Motivational variables in second language acquisition", *Canadian Journal of Psychology* Vol. 13, 266–272.

Gardner R. – Lambert W. (1972): *Attitudes and motivation: Second language learning*. Newbury House.

Gardner R. – MacIntyre P. (1991): "An instrumental motivation in language study: Who says it isn't effective?", *Studies in Second Language Acquisition* 13, 57–72.

Garrett N. (2009): "Computer-Assisted Language Learning trends and issues revisited: Integrating innovation", *The Modern Language Journal* Volume 93, Issue Supplement 1, 719–740.

Garrison D. (1997): "Self-directed learning: Toward a comprehensive model", *Adult Education Quarterly* 48, 18–33.

Gaved M. – Kukulska-Hulme A. – Jones A. – Scanlon E. – Dunwell I. – Lameras P. – Akiki O. (2013): "Creating coherent incidental learning journeys on mobile devices through feedback and progress indicators". Available at: http://oro.open.ac.uk/37816/ (date of access: 14 November 2014).

Gaved M. – P. Luley – S. Efremidis – Georgiou I. – Kukulska-Hulme A. – Jones A. – Scanlon E. (2014): "Challenges in context-aware mobile language learning: the MASELTOV approach", Available at: http://oro.open.ac.uk/40758/1/GavedM-mlearn2014-reviewed-final.pdf (date of access 20 December 2015).

Geddes S. (2004): "Mobile learning in the 21st century: Benefit to learners". Available at: http://knowledgetree.flexiblelearning.net.au/edition06/download/geddes.pdf (date of access: 15 November 2015).

Ghadirli H. – Rastgarpour M. (2012): "An adaptive and intelligent tutor by expert systems for mobile devices", *International Journal of Managing Public Sector Information and Communication Technologies (IJMPICT)* Vol. 3 No. 1. Available at: doi:10.5121/ijmpict.2012.3102 (date of access: 15 November 2015).

Ghahremani-Ghajar S. – Mohammadi Doostdar H.– Mirhosseini S. (2012): "We have been living with this pain: Enquiry based language learning in Iranian higher education", *Teaching in Higher Education* Vol. 17 No. 3, 269–281.

Geser H. (2004): "Towards a sociology of the mobile phone", *Sociology in Switzerland: Sociology of the Mobile Phone*. Available at: http://socio.ch/mobile/t_geser1.pdf (date of access: 15 November 2015).

Giddens A. (1979): *Central problems in social theory: Action, structure and contradiction in social analysis*. Berkeley: University of California Press.

Giddens A. (1984): *The constitution of society*. Cambridge: Polity Press.

Giles H. – St. Clair R. (eds.) (1979): *Language and social psychology*. Oxford: Basil Blackwell.

Gimeno S. (ed.) (2010): *New trends in Computer-Assisted Language Learning: Working together*. Gandia: Macmillan ELT.

Glendinning E. – Holmström B. (2005): *English in Medicine. 3rd ed*. Cambridge: Cambridge University Press.

Glendinning E. – Howard R. (2007): *Profesionnal English in Use: Medicine*. Cambridge: Cambridge University Press.

Global Minimum Essential Requirements in Medical Education (GMER) (2014): Available at: http://www.iime.org/documents/assessment.htm (date of access: 15 September 2014).

Godman A. (1976): "The language of science from the viewpoint of the writer of science textbooks", in J. Richards (ed.), 71–79.

Good T. – Brophy J. (1994): *Looking in classrooms (6th ed.)*. New York: HarperCollins.

Gotti M. – Salager-Meyer F. (2006): *Advances in medical discourse analysis: Written and oral contexts*. Bern: Peter Lang.

Górnicz M. (1997): "Sposoby i granice kompresji terminów", *Poradnik Językowy* (2), 25–32.

Górnicz M. (2013): "Teaching medical translation to non-medical students – a case study with some theoretical insights", *JAHR* Vol. 4 No. 7, 129–144.

Grabowski Ł. (2015): *Phraseology in English Pharmaceutical Discourse: A Corpus-Driven Study of Register Variation*. Opole: Wydawnictwo Uniwersytetu Opolskiego.

Graddol D. – Meinhof U. (eds.) (1999): *English in a changing world*. Oxford: Catchline/AILA.

Green D. – Lepper M. (1974): "How to turn play into work", *Psychology Today*, 49–54.

Greenhall S. (1981): "First experiment in designing ESP courses", *Recherches et Echanges* 6(2), 11–20.

Grucza F. (1991): *Teoretyczne podstawy terminologii*. Wrocław: Zakład Narodowy im. Ossolińskich.

Grucza S. (2013)a: *Od lingwistyki tekstu do lingwistyki tekstu specjalistycznego. Studi@ Naukowe 2*. Warsaw: Wydawnictwo Naukowe Instytutu Kulturologii i Lingwistyki Antropocentrycznej Uniwersytetu Warszawskiego.

Grucza S. (2013)b: *Lingwistyka języków specjalistycznych. Studi@ Naukowe 3.* Warsaw: Wydawnictwo Naukowe Instytutu Kulturologii i Lingwistyki Antropocentrycznej Uniwersytetu Warszawskiego.

Gulek J. – Demirtas H. (2005): "Learning with technology: The impact of laptop use on student achievement", *Journal of Technology, Learning and Assessment* 3(2), 1–39.

Hall M. – Elliott K. (2003): "Diffusion of technology into the teaching process: Strategies to encourage faculty members to embrace the laptop environment", *Journal of Education for Business* 78(6), 301–307.

Halliday M. (1993): "Some grammatical problems in scientific English", in M. Halliday – J. Martin (eds.), 69–85.

Halliday M. – Martin J. (eds.) (1993): *Writing science.* London: The Falmer Press.

Hampel R. (2009): "Teaching languages in online environments: Fostering interaction and collaboration", *Innovation in Language Learning and Teaching* 3(1), 35–50.

Hansson T. (ed.) (2008): *Handbook of research on digital information technologies: Innovations, methods and ethical issues.* Hershey: Information Science Reference.

Harper D. (ed.) (1986): "ESP for the University", *ELT Documents 123.* Oxford: Pergamon Press.

Hegedűs A. (2013): "Approaches to scoring translation in the PROFEX EMP exam", *Acta Medica Marisiensis* 59(2), 104–106.

Heift T. (2002): "Learner control and error correction in ICALL: Browsers, peekers, and adamants", *CALICO Journal* 19(2), 295–313.

Herbert A. (1965): *The structure of technical English. London: Longman Group Ltd.*

Herrington A. (2009): "Using a smartphone to create digital teaching episodes as resources in adult education", in J. Herrington – A. Herrington – J. Mantei – I. Olney – B. Ferry (eds.), 28–35.

Herrington J. – Herrington A. (2007): "Authentic mobile learning in higher education". Paper Presented at the AARE Annual Conference, Freemantle.

Herrington J. – Herrington A. – Mantei J. (2009)a: "Design principles for mobile learning", in Herrington J. – Herrington A. – Mantei J. – Olney I. – Ferry B. (eds.), 129–138.

Herrington J. – Herrington A. – Mantei – Olney I. – Ferry B. (2009)b: "Using mobile technologies to develop new ways of teaching and learning", in J. Herrington – A. Herrington – Mantei J. – Olney I. – Ferry B. (eds.), 1–14.

Herrington J. – Herrington A. – Mantei J. – Olney I. – Ferry B. (eds.) (2009): New technologies, new pedagogies: Mobile learning in higher education. Wollongong: University of Wollongong. Available at: http://ro.uow.edu.au/newtech (date of access: 15 November 2015).

Higgins J. (1967) "Hard facts: Notes on teaching English to science students", *English Language Teaching Journal* 21(1), 55–60.

Hoedt J. – Turner R. (eds.), (1981): *New bearings in LSP*. Copenhagen: The LSP Centre, UNESCO ALSED LSP Network and Newsletter, Copenhagen School of Economics.

Hoekje B. – Tipton S. (eds.) (2011): *English language and the medical profession: Instructing and assessing the communication skills of international physicians.* Bingley: Emerald Group Publishing.

Hoffman L. (1981): "The linguistic analysis and teaching of LSP in the German Democratic Republic", in Hoedt J. – Turner R. (eds.), 107–130.

Holden S. (ed.) (1977): *English for Specific Purposes.* London: Modern English Publications.

Hoppe U. (2006): "How can we integrate mobile devices with broader educational scenarios?", in M. Sharples (ed.), 31–34.

Horn B. – Stroller F. – Robinson M. (2008): "Interdisciplinary collaboration: Two heads are better than one", *English Teaching Forum* 46, 2–13.

Huang Z. (1999): "The impact of globalization on English in Chinese universities", in D. Graddol – U. Meinhof (eds.), 79–86.

Hubbard P. (2013) "Making a case for learner training in technology enhanced language learning environments", *CALICO Journal* 30(2), 163–178.

Hubbard P. – Schulz M. – Smith B. (eds.) (2013): *Learner-computer interaction in language education: A festschrift in honor of Robert Fischer.* San Marcos: CALICO.

Hulstijn J. (2001): "Intentional and incidental second language vocabulary learning: A reappraisal of elaboration, rehearsal and automaticity", in P. Robinson (ed.), 258–286.

Hung H. – Tsai J. – Chen P. (2010): "Temporal conjunctions in medical case presentations: Examples from case presentations by native and Taiwanese physicians", *The International Journal of Interdisciplinary Social Sciences* Vol. 5 No. 2, 255–263.

Hunt J. (1965): "Intrinsic motivation and its role in psychological development", in D. Levine (ed.), 189–282.

Hunter K. (1991): *Doctor's stories: The narrative structure of medical knowledge.* Princeton: Princeton University Press.

Hussin V. (2002): "An ESP program for students of nursing", in T. Orr (ed.), 25–39.

Hutchinson T. – Waters A. (1980): "ESP at the crossroads". *English for Specific Purposes (Newsletter)* 36, 1–6.

Hutchinson T. – Waters A. (1987): *English for Specific Purposes: A learning-centred approach.* Cambridge: Cambridge University Press.

Hyland K. (1998): *Hedging in scientific research articles.* Amsterdam, Philadelphia: John Benjamins.

Hyland K. (2002): "Genre: Language, context and literacy", *Annual Review of Applied Linguistics* 22, 113–135.

Hyland K. (2006)a: "Medical Discourse: Hedges", in K. Brown (ed.), 694–697.

Hyland K. (2006) b: *English for Academic Purposes. An advanced resource book.* Abingdon, New York: Routledge.

Hyland K. (2007): "Is there an 'Academic Vocabulary'?", *TESOL Quarterly* Vol. 41 No. 2, 235–253.

Hymes D. (1974): *Foundations in sociolinguistics: An ethnographic approach.* Philadephia: University of Pennsylvania Press.

Hyon S. (1996): "Genre in three traditions: Implications for ESL", *TESOL Quarterly* 30, 693–722.

Ingleton C. – Kiley M. – Cannon R. – Rogers T. (2000): "Leap into… Student-centred learning". Adelaide: The University of Adelaide. Available at: https://www.imt.liu.se/en/edu/Bologna/SCL/StudentCentredLearning.pdf (date of access: 15 November 2015).

Jacoby S. – McNamara T. (1999): "Locating competence", *English for Specific Purposes* 18(3), 213–241.

Jones A. – Issroff K. – Scanlon E. (with P. McAndrew and G. Clough) (2006): "Affective factors in learning with mobile devices", in M. Sharples, 15–20.

Johns A. (2013): "The history of English for Specific Purposes research", in: B. Paltridge – S. Starfield (eds.), 5–30.

Johns A. – Paltridge B. – Belcher D. (2011): "Introduction: New directions for ESP research", in D. Belcher – A. Johns – B. Paltridge (eds.), 1–4.

Johns, A. – Price-Machado D. (2001): "English for Specific Purposes: Tailoring courses to student needs – and to the outside world" in M. Celce-Murcia (ed.), 43–55.

Kanoksilapathan B. (2007): "Rhetorical moves in biochemistry research articles", in D. Biber – U. Connor – T. Upton (eds.), 73–119.

Keller J. (2008): "First principles of motivation to learn and e-learning", *Distance Education* 29(2), 175–185.

Kelley H. – Michela J. (1980): "Attribution theory and research", *Annual Review of Psychology* 31, 457–501.

Kennedy G. – Dalgarno B. – Bennett J. – Gray K. – Chang R. (2008): Immigrants and natives: Investigating differences between staff and students' use of technology. In Hello! Where are you in the landscape of educational technology? Proceedings of ascilite Melbourne 2008. Available at: http://www.ascilite.org.au/conferences/melbourne08/procs/kennedy.pdf (date of access: 15 November 2015).

Kennedy C. – Levy M. (2008): "L'italiano al telefonino: Using SMS to support beginners' language learning", *ReCALL Journal* 20(3), 315–330. Available at: doi:10.1017/S0958344008000530 (date of access: 15 November 2015).

Kiernan P. – Aizawa K. (2004): "Cell phones in task based learning: Are cell phones useful language learning tools?", *ReCALL* 16(1), 71–84.

Kikuchi K. (2015): *Demotivation in second language acquisition.* Bristol: Multilingual Matters.

Kim S. – Mims C. – Holmes K. (2006): "An introduction to current trends and benefits of mobile wireless technology use in higher education", *AACE Journal* 14(1), 77–100.

Kincaid J – Fishburne R. – Rogers R. – Chissom B. (1975): "Derivation of new readability formulas (automated readability index, fog count, and flesch reading ease formula) for Navy enlisted personnel", Research Branch Report 8–75.

Klopfer E. – Squire K. – Jenkins H. (2002): "Environmental detectives: PDA as a window into a virtual simulated world", Proceedings of the IEEE, 2–5.

Kommers P. – Richards G. (eds.), (2005): Proceedings of *ED-MEDIA 2005. Norfolk VA: AACE.*

Komorowska H. (2005): *Metodyka nauczania języków obcych.* Warszaw: Fraszka Edukacyjna.

Krashen S. (1985): *The input hypothesis.* London: Longman.

Krickova Z. - Polackova G. (2010): "Meeting ESP needs of nursing students at university level: Theory and practice of ESP language teaching in nursing students at Jessenius Faculty of Medicine in Martin Sloavakia", *The International Journal of Interdisciplinary Social Sciences* Vol. 5 No. 5, 219–226.

Kukulska-Hulme A. (2000): "Communication with users: Insights from second language acquisition", *Interacting with Computers* 12(6), 587–599.

Kukulska-Hulme A. (2005): "Reading course materials in e-book form and on mobile devices", in A. Kukulska-Hulme – Traxler J. (eds.), 125–132.

Kukulska-Hulme A. (2006): "Mobile usability and user experience", in A. Kukulska-Hulme – J. Traxler (eds.), 45–56.

Kukulska-Hulme A. (2007): “Mobile usability in educational contexts: What have we learnt?”, *International Review of Research in Open and Distance Learning* 8(2), 1–16.

Kukulska-Hulme A. (2008)a: “Human factors and innovation with mobile devices”, in T. Hansson (ed.), 392–403.

Kukulska-Hulme A. (2008)b: “Encyclopedic knowledge in the mobile age”, in G. Needham – A. Mohamed (eds.), 29–36.

Kukulska-Hulme A. (2008)c: “What should we do with Jack-in-the-box? Anticipating surprises in mobile learning”, in M. Allegra – A. Fulantelli – M. Gentile – D. Taibi (eds.), 7–18.

Kukulska-Hulme A. (2009)a: “Conclusions: Future directions in researching mobile learning”, in G. Vavoula – N. Pachler – A. Kukulska-Hulme (eds.), 353–365.

Kukulska-Hulme A. (2009)b: “Will mobile learning change language learning?”, *ReCALL* 21(2), 157–165.

Kukulska-Hulme A. (2010)a: *Mobile learning for quality education and social inclusion.* UNESCO Institute for Information Technologies in Education, Moscow, Russian Federation. Available at: http://oro.open.ac.uk/31256/ (date of access: 10 December 2015).

Kukulska-Hulme A. (2010)b: “Mobile learning as a catalyst for change”, *Open Learning: The Journal of Open and Distance Learning* 25(3), 181–185.

Kukulska-Hulme A. (2010)c: “Charting unknown territory: Models of participation in mobile language learning”, *International Journal of Mobile Learning and Organisation* 4(2), 116–129.

Kukulska-Hulme A. (2010)d: “*Mobile Learning: Using portable technologies to create new learning*”, *Special Issue of Open Learning* Vol. 25 Issue 3, *181–185.*

Kukulska-Hulme A. (2010)e: “Learning cultures on the move: where are we heading?”, *Journal of Educational Technology and Society* 13(4), 4–14.

Kukulska-Hulme A. (2012)a: “Language learning defined by time and place: A framework for next generation designs”, in J. Díaz-Vera (ed.), 1–13.

Kukulska-Hulme A. (2012)b: “Smart devices or people? A mobile learning quandary”, *International Journal of Learning and Media* 4(3–4), 73–77.

Kukulska-Hulme A. (2012)c: “How should the higher education workforce adapt to advancements in technology for teaching and learning?”, *The Internet and Higher Education* 15(4), 247–254.

Kukulska-Hulme A. (2013)a: “Re-skilling language learners for a mobile world”. Monterey: The International Research Foundation for English Language

Education. Available at: http://www.tirfonline.org/english-in-the-workforce/mobile-assisted-language-learning/ (date of access: 15 November 2015).

Kukulska-Hulme A. (2013)b: "Mobile learners: Who are they and who will they become?", in Z. Berge – L. Muilenburg (eds.), 145–154.

Kukulska-Hulme A. (2013)c: "Mobile-assisted language learning", in C. Chapelle (ed.), 3701–3709.

Kukulska-Hulme A. (2014): "Mobile, wearable, companionable: Emerging technological challenges and incentives for learning", *Jogos e Mobile Learning*, 12–15.

Kukulska-Hulme A. – de los Arcos B. (2011) "Triumphs and frustrations of self-motivated language learners using mobile devices", in The CAL Conference 2011 – Learning Futures: Education, Technology & Sustainability.

Kukulska-Hulme A. – de los Arcos B. (2015) "Language as a bridge connecting formal and informal language learning through mobile devices", in L. Wong, – M. Milrad – M. Specht (eds.), 281–294.

Kukulska-Hulme A. – Bull S. (2008): "Theoretical perspectives on mobile language learning diaries and noticing for learners, teachers and researchers", Proceedings of the mLearn 2008 Conference, Ironbridge Gorge, Shropshire, UK. Available at: http://oro.open.ac.uk/15105/2/384A7259.pdf (date of access: 15 November 2015).

Kukulska-Hulme A. – Bull S. (2009): "Theory-based support for mobile language learning: Noticing and recording", *International Journal of Interactive Mobile Technologies* 3(2), 12–18.

Kukulska-Hulme A. – Gaved M. – Paletta L. (2015)a: "Mobile incidental learning to support the inclusion of recent immigrants". 11th International Conference on Technology, Knowledge and Society: Big Data and the Politics of Participation in the Digital Age, University of California, Berkeley. Available at: http://oro.open.ac.uk/id/eprint/41642 (date of access: 20 October 2015).

Kukulska-Hulme A. – Jones C. (2011): "The next generation: Design and the infrastructure for learning in a mobile and networked world", in A. Olofsson – J. Lindberg (eds.), 57–78.

Kukulska-Hulme A. – Norris L. – Donohue J. (2015)b: *Mobile pedagogy for English language teaching: A guide for teachers.* London: British Council.

Kukulska-Hulme A. – Pettit J. (2007): "Self-service education: Smartphones as a catalyst for informal collective and individual learning", Mlearn '07 mobile learning conference, Melbourne, Australia. Available at: http://oro.open.ac.uk/16621/2/mLearn2007_AKH%26amp;JP.pdf (date of access: 15 November 2015).

Kukulska-Hulme A. – Pettit J. (2008): "Semi-formal learning communities for professional development in mobile learning", *Journal of Computing in Higher Education* 20(2), 35–47.

Kukulska-Hulme A. – Pettit J. (2009): "Practitioners as innovators: Emergent practice in personal mobile teaching, learning, work and leisure", in A. Mohamed (ed.), 135–155.

Kukulska-Hulme A. – Pettit J. – Bradley L. – Carvalho A. – Herrington A. – Kennedy D. – Walker A. (2009)a: "An international survey of mature students' uses of mobile devices in life and learning". Proceedings of 8th World Conference on Mobile and Contextual Learning, Orlando, Florida. Available at: http://oro.open.ac.uk/23409/ (date of access: 10 September 2015).

Kukulska-Hulme A. – Pettit J. – Bradley L. – Carvalho A. – Herrington A. – Kennedy D. – Walker A. (2011)a: "Mature students using mobile devices in life and learning", *International Journal of Mobile and Blended Learning* 3(1), 18–52. Available at: doi: 10.4018/jmbl.2011010102 (date of access: 23 September 2015).

Kukulska-Hulme A. – Sharples M. (2016): "Waypoints along learning journeys in a mobile world", in W. Ng – T. Cumming (eds.), 43–56.

Kukulska-Hulme A. – Sharples M. – Milrad M. – Arnedillo -Sánchez I. – Vavoula G. (2009)b: "Innovation in mobile learning: A European perspective", *International Journal of Mobile and Blended Learning* 1(1), 13–35.

Kukulska-Hulme A. – Sharples M. – Milrad M. – Arnedillo -Sánchez I. – Vavoula G. (2011)b: "The genesis and development of mobile learning in Europe", in D. Parsons (ed.), 151–177.

Kukulska-Hulme A. – Shield L. (2008): "An overview of mobile assisted language learning: From content delivery to supported collaboration and interaction", *ReCALL* 20(3), 271–289.

Kukulska-Hulme A. – Shield L. – Hassan X. (2010): "Mobile technologies for language learning and teaching: An exploratory investigation", in S. Gimeno (ed.), 167–174.

Kukulska-Hulme A. – Traxler J. (2007): "Designing for mobile and wireless learning", in H. Beetham – R. Sharpe (eds.), 180–192.

Kukulska-Hulme A. – Traxler J. – Petit J. (2007): "Designed and user-generated activity in the mobile age", *Journal of Learning Design* 2(1), 52–65.

Kukulska-Hulme A. – Traxler J. (eds.) (2005): Mobile learning: A handbook for educators and trainers. London and New York: Routledge.

Kukulska-Hulme A. – Wible D. (2008): "Context at the crossroads of language learning and mobile learning", ICCE 2008 Workshop Proceedings, Taiwan.

Available at: http://oro.open.ac.uk/13053/1/workshop_paper1.pdf (date of access: 20 October 2015).

Kuo C. (2005): "Wireless technology in higher education: The perceptions of faculty and students concerning the use of wireless laptops". Available at: https://etd.ohiolink.edu/!etd.send_file?accession=ohiou1125521504&disposition=inline (date of access: 20 September 2015).

Kuźmicz K. – Skrzydlewski W. (2012): "Metodologiczny kontekst badania e-learningu", in W. Skrzydlewski – S. Dylak (eds.), 81–102.

Labov J. – Hanau C. (2011): "Pronunciation as life and death: Improving the communication skills of non-native English speaking pathologists" in Barbara J. Hoekje – Sara Tipton (eds.), 261–285.

Lackstrom J. – Selinker L. – Trimble L. (1972): "Grammar and technical English", *English Teaching Forum* 10 (5), 3–14.

Lamb T. – Reinders H. (2005): "Learner independence in language teaching: A concept of change", in D. Cunningham – A. Hatoss (eds.), 225–239.

Lamb T. – Reinders H. (eds.) (2008): *Learner and teacher autonomy: concepts, realities and responses*. Amsterdam: John Benjamin.

Landauer T. – Bjork R. (1978): "Optimum rehearsal patterns and name learning", in M. Gruneberg – P. Morris – R. Sykes (eds.), 625–632.

Lane C. – Yamashiro G. (2008): "Assessing learning and scholarly technologies: Lessons from an institutional survey", *Educause Quarterly* 31(3), 1–8.

Larsen-Freeman D. (2003): *Teaching language: From grammar to grammaring*. Boston: Thomson Heinle.

Larson J. (2009): *Educational psychology: Cognition and learning, individual differences and motivation*. New York: Nova Science Publishers, Inc.

Laurillard D. (2002): *Rethinking university teaching: A conversational framework for the effective use of learning technologies*. London: Routledge Falmer.

Laurillard D. (2007): "Pedagogical forms for mobile learning", in N. Pachler (ed.), 153–175.

Leaver, B. – M. Ehrman – Shekhtman B. (2005): *Achieving success in second language acquisition*. Cambridge: Cambridge University Press.

Lee M. – McLoughlin C. (eds.) (2011): *Web 2.0-Based e-Learning: Applying social informatics for tertiary teaching*. Hershey, New York: IGI Global.

Lefoe G. – Olney I. – Wright R. – Herrington A. (2009): "Faculty development for new technologies: Putting mobile learning in the hands of the teachers", in J. Herrington – A. Herrington – J. Mantei – I. Olney – B. Ferry (eds.), 15–27.

Leibling M. – Prior R. (2005): *The A-Z of learning. Tips and techniques for teachers*. Abingdon, New York: Routledge Falmer.

Leitner S. (1972): *So lernt man lernen. Angewandte Lernpsychologie – ein Weg zum Erfolg*. Freiburg im Breisgau. Verlag, Herder.

Lepper M. – Keavney M. – Drake M. (1996): "Intrinsic motivation and extrinsic rewards", *Review of Educational Research* 66(1), 5–32.

Leung L. – Wei R. (2000): More than just talk on the move: A use-and-gratification study of the cellular phone. *Journalism & Mass Communication Quarterly* 77(2), 308–320.

Levine, D. (ed.) (1965): *Nebraska symposium on motivation* Vol. 13. Lincoln: University of Nebraska Press.

Li L. – Ge G. (2009): Genre analysis: Structural and linguistic evolution of the English-medium medical research article (1985–2004)", *English for Specific Purposes* 28: 93–104.

Liaw S. (2008): "Investigating students' perceived satisfaction, behavioral intention, and effectiveness of e-learning: A case study of the Blackboard system", *Computers & Education* 51, 864–873.

Lightbown P. – Spada N. (1993): *How languages are learned*. Oxford: OUP.

Lindemann, S. – Mauranen A. (2001): "'It's just real messy': The occurrence and function of just in a corpus of academic speech", *English for Specific Purposes* 20, Supplement 1, 459–475.

Little D. (1993): "Autonomy in language learning: Some theoretical and practical considerations", in A. Swarbrick (ed.), 81–87.

Little D. (1995): "Learning as dialogue: the dependence of learner autonomy on teacher autonomy", *System* 23(2), 175–181.

Little D. (1997): "Language awareness and the autonomous language learner", *Language Awareness* 6,(2–3), 93–104.

Little D. (2007)a: "Language learner autonomy: Some fundamental considerations revisited", *Innovation in Language Learning and Teaching* 1(1), 14–29.

Little D. (2007)b: "Introduction: Reconstructing learner and teacher autonomy in language education", in A. Barfield – S. Brown (eds.), 1–12.

Little D. (2008): "Learner autonomy in practice: A challenge for university language teaching", in R. Arntz – B. Kühn (eds.), 47–63.

Little D. (2009)a: "Learner autonomy, the European Language Portfolio and teacher development", in R. Pemberton – S. Toogood – A. Barfield (eds.), 147–173.

Little D. (2009)b: "Language learner autonomy and the European Language Portfolio: Two L2 English examples", *Language Learning* 42(2), 222–233.

Liu J. (2013): "Using Facebook for learning writing: EFL students' perceptions and challenges", Paper presented at the 30th International Conference on English Teaching and Learning, Tainan, Taiwan.

Locke E. – Latham G. (1990): *A theory of goal setting and task performance.* Upper Saddle River: Prentice Hall.

Loiacono A. (2013) "Sociomedical interaction in English: Towards virtual hospital", *JAHR* Vol. 4 No. 7, 195–215.

Long M. (ed.) (2005): *Second language needs analysis.* Cambridge: CUP.

Long M. – Crookes G. (1992): "Three approaches to task-based syllabus design", *Teaching English to Speakers of Other Languages Quarterly* 26(1), 27–56.

Lores R. (2004): "On RA abstracts: from rhetorical structure to thematic organization", *English for Specific Purposes* 23, 280–302.

Lu M. (2008): "Effectiveness of vocabulary learning via mobile phone", *Journal of Computer Assisted Learning* 24(6), 515–525.

Lukmani Y. (1972): "Motivation to learn and language proficiency", *Language Learning* 22, 261–274.

Łukasik M. (ed.) (2008): *Debiuty Naukowe II. Terminologia-translatoryka-terminografia.* Warsaw: Katedra Języków Specjalistycznych Wydział Lingwistyki Stosowanej i Filologii Wschodniosłowiańskich Uniwersytetu Warszawskiego.

Ma M. – Oliveira M. – Petersen S. – Hauge J. (eds.), (2013): Serious games development and applications. Proceedings of 4th International Conference, SGDA 2013, Trondheim: Springer.

Mac Callum K. (2009): "Student characteristics and variables that determine mobile learning adoption: An initial study". Proceedings of the Universal College of Learning: Teaching and Learning Conference, Palmerston North, NZ. Available at: http://akoaotearoa.ac.nz/download/ng/file/group-3740/n3750-student-characteristics-and-variablesthat-determine-mobile-learning-adoption---an-initial-study---mac callum.pdf (date of access: 15 July 2015).

Mac Callum K. – Jeffrey L. (2009): "Identifying discriminating variables that determine mobile learning adoption by educators: An initial study", in R. Atkinson – C. McBeath (eds.), 602–608.

Mackiewicz J. (2004): "The effects of tutor expertise in engineering writing: A linguistic analysis of writing tutors' comments", *IEEE Transactions on Professional Communication* 47, 316–329.

Maher J. (1986): "The development of English as an international language of medicine", *Applied Linguistics* 7, 206–218.

Malcolm L. (1987): "What rules govern tense usage in scientific articles?", *English for Specific Purposes* 6, 31–44.

Malone T. (1981): "Toward a theory of intrinsically motivating instruction", *Cognitive Science 4,* 333–370.

Manning A. – Martin P. – McCalla K. (eds.) (1983): The Tenth LACUS Forum.

Marcos L. – Hilera J. – Barchino R. – Jiménez L. – Martínez J. – Gutiérrez J. – J. Gutiérrez – Otón S. (2010): "An experiment for improving students performance in secondary and tertiary education by means of m-learning auto-assessment", *Computers & Education* 55, 1069–1079.

Martin A. (1976): "Teaching academic vocabulary to foreign graduate students", *TESOL Quarterly* 10 (1), 91–99.

Martin A. (2006): *Building classroom success. Eliminating academic fear and failure.* London, New York: Continuum.

Martin R. – McGill T. – Sudweeks F. (2013): "Learning anywhere, anytime: Student motivators for m-learning", *Journal of Information Technology Education: Research* Vol. 12, 51–67. Available at: http://www.jite.org/documents/Vol12/JITEv12ResearchP051-067MartinFT51.pdf (date of access: 21 September 2015).

Martín-Monje E. – Arús J. – Rodríguez-Arancón P. – Calle-Martínez C. (2013): "REALL: rubric for the evaluation of apps in language learning". Available at: http://eprints.ucm.es/25096/1/Rubric%20for%20the%20Evaluation%20of%20Apps%20in%20Language%20Learning.pdf (date of access: 21 October 2015).

Maslow A. (1970): *Motivation and personality. Second edition.* New York: Harper & Row.

McClelland D. (1965): "Achievement and entrepreneurship: A longitudinal study", *Journal of Personality & Social Psychology* 1, 389–393.

McClelland D. (2000): "Goal orientations in Japanese college students learning EFL", in S. Cornwell – P. Robinson (eds.), 99–115.

McCombs S. – Liu Y. (2006) "Turning iPod into an effective portable learning tool", in C. Crawford – D. Willis – R. Carlsen – I. Gibson – K. McFerrin – J. Price – R. Weber (eds.), 438–443.

McCombs S. – Pope J. (1994)*: *Motivating hard to reach students.* Washington: American Psychological Association.

McDonough S. (1986): *Psychology in foreign language teaching. Second edition.* London: Allen & Unwin.

McLean N. (2003): *The M-learning paradigm: An overview.* Royal Academy of Engineering and the Vodafone Group Foundation.

McMillan K. – Honey M. (1993): Year one of project pulse: Pupils using laptops in science and English. A final report. New York: Center for Technology in

Education. Available at: http://files.eric.ed.gov/fulltext/ED358822.pdf (date of access: 17 August 2015).

McNicholl J. (2005): "Language e-learning on the move", *Japan Media Review*. Available at: http://ojr.org/ japan/wireless/1080854640.php (date of access: 23 November 2014).

Miller M. – Piller M. (2005): "Principal factors of an audio reading delivery mechanism: Evaluating educational use of the iPod", in P. Kommers – G. Richards (eds.), 2581–2588.

Milrad M. (2006): "How should learning activities using mobile technologies be designed to support innovative educational practices?", in M. Sharples, 28–30.

Mintz D. (1992): "What's in a word: The distancing function of language in medicine", *The Journal of Medical Humanities* 13, 223–233.

Mioduser D. – Nachmias R. – Oren A. – Lahav O. (1999): "Web-based learning environments: Current states and emerging trends", in B. Collis – R. Oliver (eds.), 753–758.

Mischler E. (1984): *The discourse of medicine: Dialectics of medical interviews*. Norwood: Ablex.

MOBILearn (2003): The mobilearn project vision. The MOBILearn Project. Available at: ftp://ftp.cordis.europa.eu/pub/ist/docs/ka3/mobilearn.pdf (date of access: 10 November 2015)

Mohan B. – Beckett G. (2003): "A functional approach to research on content-based language learning: Recasts in causal explanations", *The Modern Language Journal* 87(3), 421–432.

Mohamed A. (2009): *Mobile Learning: Transforming the delivery of education and training. Issues in Distance Education*. Athabasca: Athabasca University Press.

Morita M. (2008): The Mobile Based Learning (MBL) in Japan. Proceedings of the First Conference on Creating, Connecting and Collaborating through Computing. Available at: http://csdl2.computer.org/comp/proceedings/c5/2003/1975/00/19750128.pdf (date of access: 20 January 2015).

Mortimer F. (1834): *Reading disentangled; or classified lessons in spelling and reading*. London: Edward Stanford.

Motiwalla L. (2007): "Mobile learning: A framework and evaluation", *Computers & Education* 49, 581–596.

Mudraya O. (2006): "Engineering English: A lexical frequency instructional model", *English for Specific Purposes* 25: 235–256.

Munby J. (1978): *Communicative syllabus design*. Cambridge: Cambridge University Press.

Murray D. (1997): "Plain English or plain confusing", *Missouri Law Review* Vol. 62 Issue 2, 345–379.

Myers G. (1985): "Text as *knowledge claims*: The *social construction* of *two biologists' articles*", *Social Studies of Science* 15(4): 593–630.

Naiman N. – Frolich M. – Stern H. – Todesco A. (1995): *The good language learner.* Clevedon: Multilingual Matters Ltd.

Naismith L. – Lonsdale P. – Vavoula G. – Sharples M. (2004): *Literature review in mobile technologies and learning.* Bristol: Futurelab.

Nation P. (2001): *Learning vocabulary in another language.* Cambridge: Cambridge university Press.

Nation P. (2008): *Teaching Vocabulary: Strategies and techniques.* Boston: Heinle Cengage.

Needham G. – Mohamed A. (eds.) (2008): *M-libraries: Libraries on the move to provide virtual access.* London: Facet Publishing.

Nesi H. (2013): "ESP and corpus studies", in B. Paltridge – S. Starfield (eds.), 407–426.

Newhouse C. (2001): "A follow-up study of students using portable computers at a secondary school", *British Journal of Educational Technology* 32(2), 209–219. Available at: doi: 10.1111/1467–8535.00191 (date of access: 14 August 2015).

Ng W. – Howard N. (2016): "Sustaining innovation in learning with mobile devices: Key challenges", in W. Ng – T. Cumming (eds.), 1–25.

Ng W. – Cumming T. (eds.) (2016): *Sustaining mobile learning: Theory, research and practice.* Abingdon, New York: Routledge. Available at: http://www.amazon.co.uk/Sustaining-Mobile-Learning-Routledge-Education/dp/1138787388 (date of access: 15 November 2015).

Nickerson C. (2013): "English for Specific Purposes and English as a Lingua Franca", in B. Paltridge – S. Starfield (eds.), 445–460.

Noels K. (2001): "New orientations in language learning motivation: Towards a model of intrinsic, extrinsic, and integrative orientations and motivation", in Z. Dörnyei – R. Schmidt (eds.), 43–68.

Noels K. (2003): "Learning Spanish as a second language: Learners' orientations and perceptions of their teachers' communication style", in Z. Dörnyei (ed.), 97–136.

Norbrook H. – Scott P. (2003): "Motivation in mobile modern foreign language learning", in J. Attewell – G. Da Bormida – M. Sharples – C. Savill-Smith (eds.), 50–51.

Nowicki W. (1978): *O ścisłość pojęć i kulturę słowa w technice.* Warsaw: Wydawnictwa Komunikacji i Łączności.

Nowicki W. (1986): *Podstawy terminologii.* Wrocław: Zakład Narodowy im. Ossolińskich.

Nyiri K. (2002): Towards a Philosophy of M-Learning. IEEE International Workshop on Wireless and Mobile Technologies in Education (WMTE 2002), Teleborg Campus.

Oberg A. – Daniels P. (2013): "Analysis of the effect a student-centred mobile learning instructional method has on language acquisition", *Computer Assisted Language Learning* 26(2), 177–196.

Oblinger D. – Oblinger J. (eds.) (2005): *Educating the Net Generation.* Boulder: EDUCAUSE. Available at: https://net.educause.edu/ir/library/pdf/pub7101.pdf (date of access: 5 September 2015).

Olofsson A. – Lindberg J. (eds.) (2011): *Informed design of educational technologies in higher education: Enhanced learning and teaching.* Hershey: Information Science Reference (an Imprint of IGI Global).

Oloruntoba R. (2006): "Mobile learning environments: A conceptual overview", in A. Brown (ed.), 1–9.

O'Malley C. – Vavoula G. – Glew J. – Taylor J. – Sharples M. – Lefrere P. (2005): *Guidelines for learning/teaching/tutoring in a mobile environment. Mobilearn project deliverable.* Available at: https://hal.archives-ouvertes.fr/hal-00696244/document (data of access: 27 February 2014).

Ong L. – de Haes J. – Hoos A. – Lammes F. (1995): "Doctor-patient communication: a review of the literature" *Social Science & Medicine* Vol. 40, 903-918.

Ophir E. – Nass C. – Wagner A. (2009): "Cognitive control in media multitaskers", *Proceedings of the National Academy of Sciences* 106(37), 15583–15587.

Orr T. (2002): "Introduction: The nature of English for Specific Purposes", in T. Orr (ed.), 1–2.

Orr T. (ed.) (2002): *English for Specific Purposes.* Alexandria: Teachers of English to Speakers of Other Languages, Inc.

Osborne J. (2009): *IELTS Research Reports Volume 10.* Canberra: IELTS Australia and British Council.

Osuna A. (1982): *En Busca de un Lexico Basico de Biolog'ia.* Unpublished PhD dissertation. University of the Andes, Merida, Venezuela.

Oxford R. – Shearin J. (1994): "Language learning motivation: Expanding the theoretical framework", *The Modern Language Journal* 78(1), 12–28.

Pachler N. (ed.) (2007): *Mobile learning: Towards a research agenda.* London, UK: WLE Centre.

Paletta L. – Dunwell I. – Gaved M. – Bobeth J. – Efremidis S. – Luley P. – Kukulska+-Hulme A. – de Freitas S. – Lameras P. – Deutsch S. (2013): "Advances in the

MASELTOV game – Mobile assistance for social inclusion and empowerment of immigrants with persuasive learning technologies and social network services". Proceedings of the 10th International Conference on Advances in Computer Entertainment (ACE 2013), Enschede, Netherlands. Available at: http://link.springer.com/chapter/10.1007%2F978-3-319-03161-3_33 (date of access: 14 October 2015).

Paltridge B. (2000): *Making sense of discourse.* Gold Coast: Antepoedean Educational Enterprises.

Paltridge B. (2002): "Thesis and dissertation writing: An examination of published advice and actual practice", *English for Specific Purposes* 21, 125–143.

Paltridge B. (2012): *Discourse* analysis. 2nd ed. London: Continuum.

Paltridge B. – Starfield S. (eds.) (2013): *The handbook of English for Specific Purposes.* Chichester: Wiley-Blackwell.

Park B. (2006): "How to increase the adoption and utilization of m-learning?" in T. Reeves – S. Yamashita (eds.), 2271–2276.

Parkinson J. (2000): "Acquiring scientific literacy through content and genre: A theme-based language course for science students", in *English for Specific Purposes* 19, 369–387.

Parkinson J. (2013): "English for Science and Technology", in B. Paltridge – S. Starfield (eds.), 155–170.

Parsons D. (ed.) (2011): *Combining e-learning and m-learning: New applications of blended educational resources.* Hershey: Information Science Reference (an imprint of IGI Global).

Patten B. – Sanchez I. – Tangney B. (2005): "Designing collaborative, constructionist and contextual applications for handheld devices", *Computers & Education* 46, 294–308.

Pearson C. – Gaved M. – Brasher A. – Jones A. – Kukulska-Hulme A. – Scanlon E. – Jones J. – Neumann L. – Busta M. (2014): *Mobile situated language learning.* Graz: MASELTOV Consortium.

Pemberton R. – Toogood S. – Barfield A. (eds.) (2009): *Maintaining control: Autonomy and language learning.* Hong Kong: Hong Kong University Press.

Perry D. (2003): *Handheld computers (PDAs) in schools.* Coventry: BECTA.

Petri H. (2003): *Motivation: Theory and research.* Belmont: Wadsworth.

Pettit J. – Kukulska-Hulme A. (2007): "Going with the grain: Mobile devices in practice", *Australasian Journal of Educational Technology* 23 (1), 17–33.

Pettit J. – Kukulska-Hulme A. (2008): "Do smart devices make smart learners?" Proceedings of the MLearn 2008 Conference. Ironbridge Gorge, Shropshire, UK.

Pettit J. – Kukulska-Hulme A. (2011): "Mobile 2.0: crossing the border into formal learning?", in M. Lee – C. McLoughlin (eds.), 192–208.

Pęcherzewska A. – Knot S. (2007): *Review of existing EU projects dedicated to dyslexia, gaming in education and m-learning.* WR08 Report to CallDysc project.

Phillips M. – Shettlesworth C. (1978): "How to *ARM your students*: A *consideration* of *two approaches* to *providing materials* for *ESP*", *English for Specific Purposes. ELT Documents 101.*

Piaget J. (1952): *The origins of intelligence in children.* New York: Norton.

Piaget J. (1972) The principles of genetic epistemology. New York: Basic Books.

Pica T. (1981): "Quelques remarques apropos des problemes poses par l'elaboration d'une theorie propre au traitement des langues de specialite", in J. Hoedt – R.Turner (eds.), 25–46.

Pimsleur P. (1967): "A memory schedule", *The Modern Language Journal* 51, 73–75.

Pinna A. (2007): "Exploiting LSP corpora in the study of foreign languages", in D. Galova (ed.), 146–162.

Pinto dos Santos V. (2002): "Genre analysis of business letters of negotiation", *English for Specific Purposes* 21(2), 167–99.

Pintrich P. (2003): "A motivational science perspective on the role of student motivation in learning and teaching contexts", *Journal of Educational Psychology* 95(4), 667–686.

Pintrich P. – Schunk D. (2002): *Motivation in education: Theory, research, and applications. 2nd ed.* Michigan: Merrill.

Pownell D. (2006): "The what, how, and why of podcasting in teacher education", in Crawford C. – Willis D. – Carlsen R. – Gibson I. – McFerrin K. – Price J. – Weber R. (eds.), 2378–2379.

Preece J. (2000): *Online communities: Designing usability, supporting sociability.* Chichester: John Wiley & Sons.

Preece J. – Rogers Y. – Sharp H. – Benyon D. – Holland S. – Carey T. (1994): *Human-Computer Interaction*. Essex: Addison-Wesley Longman Limited.

Presson N. – Davy C. – MacWhitnney B. (2013): "Experimentalized CALL for adult second language learners", in Schwieter J. (ed.), 139–164.

Proctor N. – Burton J. (2003): Tate Modern multimedia tour pilots. MLEARN 2003: Learning with mobile devices. London: LSDA, 54–55.

Puppel S. (2012): "Remarks on learner autonomy and success in foreign language learning as a measure of learner resilience", *GLOTTODIDACTICA* XXXIX, 7–12.

Quirk R. – Greenbaum S. – Leech G. – Svartik J. (1972): *A grammar of contemporary English.* London: Longman.

Quinn C. (2000): "Mlearning: Mobile, wireless, in your pocket learning. *Linezine* 2000" Available at: http://linezine.com/2.1/features/cqmmwiyp.htm (date of access: 10 June 2012).

Qvistgaard J. (1981): "La *place* des *langues* de *spécialité* (LSP) dans l'enseignement des langues vivantes", in J. Hoedt – R. Turner (eds.), 143–150.

Randall M. (2007): *Memory, psychology, and second language learning: Learning language and language teaching.* Amsterdam: John Benjamins.

Rau P. – Gao Q. – Wu L. (2008): "Using mobile communication technology in high school education: Motivation, pressure, and learning performance", *Computers & Education* 50, 1–22.

Read J. (2007): "Second language vocabulary assessment", *International Journal of English Studies* 7, 105–125.

Read J. – Wette R. (2009): "Achieving English proficiency for professional registration: The experience of overseas-qualified health professionals in the New Zealand context", In J. Osborne (ed.), 181–222. Available at: http://hdl.handle.net/2292/13601 (date of access: 10 December 2015).

Rees J. – Pattison J. – Williams G. (2007): *100 cases in clinical medicine. 2nd edition.* Boca Raton: Taylor & Francis Group, LLC.

Reeves T. – Yamashita S. (eds.), (2006): Proceedings of World Conference on E-Learning in Corporate, Government, Healthcare, and Higher Education. Chesapeake: AACE.

Reinders H. – Hubbard P. (2013): "CALL and learner autonomy: Affordances and constraints", in M. Thomas – Reinders H. – Warschauer M. (eds.). 359–375.

Ribes R. – Aranda P. – Giba J. (2010): *Surgical English.* Berlin: Springer.

Richards J. – Rogers T. (1986): *Approaches and methods in language teaching: A description and analysis.* Cambridge: CUP.

Richards J. (ed.) (1976): *Teaching English for Science and Technology.* Regional English Language Centre: Singapore University Press.

Roberts G. (2005): "Technology and learning expectations of the Net Generation" in Oblinger D. – Oblinger J. (eds.), 3.1–3.7.

Robinson P. (1980): *ESP (English for Specific Purposes).* Oxford: Pergamon.

Robinson P. (1991): *ESP today: A practitioner's guide.* Hemel Hampstead: Prentice-Hall.

Robinson P. (ed.) (2001): *Cognition and second language instruction.* Cambridge: Cambridge University Press.

Roblyer M. – Doering A. (2010): *Integrating educational technology into teaching. 5th ed.* New York: Allyn & Bacon.

Rogers S. (2007): *Mastering scientific and medical writing. A self-help guide.* Berlin, Heidelberg, New York: Springer.

Rogers Y. – Price S. – Stanton F. – Randell C. – Weal M. – Fitzpatrick G. (2005): "Ubi-learning integrates indoor and outdoor experiences", *Communications of the ACM*, 48(1), 55–59.

Rose K – Kasper G. (eds.) (2001): *Pragmatics in language teaching.* Cambridge: Cambridge University Press.

Roter D. – Hall J. (1989): "Studies of doctor-patient interaction", *Annu Rev Public Health* 10, 163–180.

Rubin J. (1975): "What the 'Good language learner' can teach us", *TESOL Quarterly* Vol. 9 No. 1, 41–51.

Rubin J. – Thompson I. (1982): *How to be a more successful language learner.* Boston: Heinle & Heinle.

Ruchter M. – Klar B. – Geiger W. (2010): "Comparing the effects of mobile computers and traditional approaches in environmental education", *Computers & Education* 54, 1054–1067.

Ruiz-Garrido M. – Palmer-Silveira J. – Fortanet-Gómez I. (eds.) (2010): *English for profession and academic purposes.* Amsterdam: Rodopi.

Salager-Meyer F. (1977): *Optimum foundations of English technical literature and their application to the comprehension training of non-English-speaking scientists.* Unpublished PhD dissertation. University of Texas at Austin.

Salager-Meyer F. (1983): "The lexis of fundamental medical English: Classificatory framework and rhetorical function (A Statistical Approach)", *Reading in a Foreign Language* Vol. 1 No. 1, 54–64.

Salager-Meyer F. (1992): "A text-type and move analysis of verb tense and modality distribution in medical English abstracts", *English for Specific Purposes* 11(2), 93–115.

Salager-Meyer F. (1994): Hedges and textual communicative function in medical English written discourse", *English for Specific Purposes* 13(2), 149-171.

Salager-Meyer F. – M. Alcaraz Ariza – Pabón Berbesí (2010): "Hidden influencers and the scholarly enterprise: A cross-linguistic/cultural analysis of acknowledgments in medical research papers", in M. Ruiz-Garrido – J. Palmer-Silveira – I. Fortanet-Gómez (eds.), 43–56.

Salager-Meyer F. – Alcaraz Ariza M. – Luzardo Briceño M. (2013): "Titling and authorship practices in medical case reports: A diachronic study (1840–2009)", *Communication and Medicine*, 63–80.

Samraj B. (2002): "Introductions in research articles: Variations across disciplines", *English for Specific Purposes* 21(1), 1–17.

Scanlon E. – Gaved M. – Jones A. – Kukulska-Hulme A. – Paletta L. – Dunwell I. (2014): "Representations of an incidental learning framework to support mobile learning". Proceedings of 10th International Conference on Mobile Learning 2014, Madrid, Spain, IADIS Press, 238–242.

Scanlon E. – Jones A. – Waycott J. (2005): "Mobile technologies: Prospects for their use in learning in informal science settings", *Journal of Interactive Media in Education, Special issue on portable learning: Experiences with mobile devices*. Available at: http://jime.open.ac.uk/articles/10.5334/2005-25/ (date of access: 15 November 2015).

Scheidecker D. – Freeman W. (1999): *Bringing out the best in students: How legendary teachers motivate kids*. London: SAGE.

Schmidmaier R. – Ebersbach R. – Schiller M. – Hege I. – Holzer M. – Fischer M. (2011) "Using electronic flashcards to promote learning in medical students: Retesting versus restudying", Med Educ. 45(11), 1101–1110. Available at: doi: 10.1111/j.1365-2923.2011.04043.x (date of access: 15 November 2015).

Schumann J. (1986): "Research on the acculturation model for second language acquisition", *Journal of Multilingual and Multicultural Development* Vol. 7 Issue 5, 379–392.

Schumann J. (2000): "Appraisal psychology, neurobiology, and language", *Annual Review of Applied Linguistics* Vol. 21, 23–42.

Schunk D. – Pintrich P. – Meece J. (2008): *Motivation in education: Theory, research, and applications. 3rd ed.* Upper Saddle River: Pearson.

Schwieter J. (ed.) (2013): *Innovative research and practice in second language acquisition and bilingualism*. Amsterdam/Philadelphia: John Benjamins Publishing Company.

Scott D. – Nishimura S. – Kato S. (2006): "Using iPods to support content area learning in a Japanese college lecture course", in T. Reeves – S. Yamashita (eds.), 3014–3019.

Seifert T. – O'Keefe B. (2001): The relationship of work avoidance and learning goals to perceived competence, externality and meaning. *British Journal of Educational Psychology* 71, 81–92.

Seta L. – Kukulska-Hulme A. – Arrigo M. (2014): "What have we learnt about mobile LifeLong Learning (mLLL)?", *International Journal of Lifelong Education* 33(2), 161–182.

Sha, L. – Looi C. – Chen W. – Zhang B. (2012) "Understanding mobile learning from the perspective of self-regulated learning", *Journal of Computer Assisted*

*Learning* 28(4), 366–378. Available at: doi: 10.1111/j.1365-2729.2011.00461.x (date of access: 15 July 2015).

Sharples M. (2000): "The design of personal mobile technologies for lifelong learning", *Computers and Education* 34, 177–193.

Sharples M. (2005): "Learning as conversation: Transforming education in the mobile age". Proceedings of Seeing, Understanding, Learning in the Mobile Age, 147–152.

Sharples M. (2006): "How can we address the conflicts between personal informal learning and traditional classroom education?", in M. Sharples (ed.), 21–24.

Sharples M. (ed.) (2006): Big issues in mobile learning. Report of a workshop by the Kaleidoscope Network of Excellence Mobile Learning Initiative, University of Nottingham, UK.

Sharples M. – Corlett D. – Westmancott O. (2002): "The design and implementation of a mobile learning resource", *Personal and Ubiquitous Computing* 6, 220–234.

Sharples, M. – Taylor J. – Vavoula G. (2007): "A theory of learning for the mobile age", in Andrews R. – Haythornthwaite C. (ed.), 221–247.

Shepherd C. (2001): *M is for maybe*. Brighton: Fastrak Consulting Ltd.

Shi L. (2009): "English for medical purposes", in D. Belcher (ed.), 205–228.

Shield L. – Kukulska-Hulme (2008): *Special issue of ReCALL on Mobile Assisted Language Learning*. Cambridge University Press.

Sitkowski K. (2008): "Kompresja w tekstach specjalistycznych", in M. Łukasik, 26–30.

Skelton J. (1997): "The representation of truth in academic medical writing", *Applied Linguistics* 18 (2): 121–140.

Skelton J. – Hobbs F. (1999): "Concordancing: The use of language-based research in medical communication", *The Lancet* 353, 108–111.

Skelton, J. – Wearn A. – Hobbs F. (2002): "'I' and 'we': A concordancing analysis of doctors and patients use first person pronouns in primary care consultations", *Family Practice* 19(5), 484–488.

Skrzydlewski W. – Dylak S. (2012): *Media – Edukacja – Kultura: W stronę edukacji medialnej*. Poznań, Rzeszów: PTTiME.

Smith M. – Kukulska-Hulme A. (2012): "Building mobile learning capacity in higher education: E-books and iPads", in M. Specht, – J. Multisilta – M. Sharples (eds.), 298–301.

Soler V. (2002): Analysing adjectives in scientific discourse: an exploratory study with educational applications for Spanish speakers at advanced university level. English for Specific Purposes, 21(2), 145–65.

Specht M. – Multisilta J. – Sharples M. (eds.) (2012): Proceedings of 11th World Conference on Mobile and Contextual Learning. Helsinki: CELSTEC & CICERO Learning.

Spolsky B. (1969): "Attitudinal aspects of second language learning", *Language Learning* 19, 271–283.

Sternberg R. – Lubart T. (1995): *Defying the crowd: Cultivating creativity in a culture of conformity*. New York: Free Press.

Stockwell G. (2007): "Vocabulary on the move: investigating an intelligent mobile phone-based vocabulary tutor", *Computer Assisted Language Learning* 20 (4): 365–383.

Stockwell G. (2010): "Using mobile phones for vocabulary activities: Examining the effect of the platform", *Language Learning & Technology* 14(2), 95–110.

Stockwell G. (2013): "Tracking learner usage of mobile phones for language learning outside of the classroom", in P. Hubbard – M. Schulz – B. Smith (eds.), 118–136.

Stockwell G. – Hubbard P. (2013): "Some emerging principles for mobile-assisted language learning". Available at: http://www.tirfonline.org/english-in-the-work-force/mobile-assisted-language-learning (date of access: 20 December 2015).

Strevens (1988): *"ESP after twenty years: A re-appraisal"* in M. Tickoo (ed.), 1–13.

Sullivan P. – Girginer H. (2002): "The use of discourse analysis to enhance ESP teacher knowledge: An example using aviation English", *English for Specific Purposes* 21(4), 397–404.

Swales J. (1971): *Writing scientific English*. Walton on Thames: Nelson.

Swales J. (1981): *Aspects of article introductions*. The Language Studies Unit: The University of Aston.

Swales J. (1985): *Episodes in ESP.* Oxford: Pergamon.

Swales J. (1988): *Episodes in ESP: A source and reference book on the development of English for science and technology. 2nd impression*. New York: Prentice Hall.

Swales J. (1990): *Genre analysis: English in academic and research settings*. Cambridge: Cambridge University Press.

Swarbrick A. (ed.) (1993): *Teaching modern languages*. London: Routledge.

Taavitsainen, I. – Pahta P. (2000): "Conventions of professional writing: The medical case report in a historical perspective", *Journal of English Linguistics* 28, 60–76.

Tang S. – Hall V. (1995): “The overjustification effect: A metaanalysis”, *Applied Cognitive Psychology* 9(5), 365–404.

Tardieu C. (2013): “Testing et certification”, *RCDL*, Vol. 10 No. 2, 237–51.

Tarone E. – Dwyer S. – Gillette S. – Icke V. (1981): “On the use of the passive in two astrophysics journal papers”, *The ESP Journal* 1(2), 123–140.

Taveira-Gomes T. – Prado-Costa R. – Severo M. – Ferreira M. (2015): “Characterization of medical students recall of factual knowledge using learning objects and repeated testing in a novel e-learning system”, *BMC Med Educ.* 24/15/4. Available at: doi: 10.1186/s12909-014-0275-0 (date of access: 15 November 2015).

Taylor R. (2005): *The clinician's guide to medical writing*. Berlin: Springer.

Thomas J. – Wilson A. (1996): “Methodologies for studying a corpus of doctor-patient interaction” in J. Thomas – M. Short (eds.), 92–109.

Thomas J. – Short M. (eds.) (1996): *Using corpora for language research*. London: Longman.

Thomas M – Reinders H. – Warschauer M. (eds.) (2013): *Contemporary computer assisted language learning*. London: Continuum Books.

Thompson P. (1999): “Exploring the context of writing: Interviews with PhD supervisors”, in P. Thompson (ed.), 37–54.

Thompson P. (ed.) (1999): Issues in EAP writing research and instruction. Reading: Centre for Applied Language Studies, University of Reading.

Thorndike E. – Lorge I. (1944): *The teacher's word book of 30,000 words*. New York: Teachers College, Columbia University, Bureau of Publications.

Thorne S. (2003): Artifacts and cultures-of-use in intercultural communication. *Language Learning & Technology*, *7*(2), 38–67.

Thornton P. – Houser C. (2005): “Using mobile phones in English education in Japan”, *Journal of Computer Assisted Learning* 21(3), 217–228.

Tickoo M. (ed.) (1988): *ESP: State of the art*. Singapore: SEAMEO Regional Centre.

Traxler J. (2005): “Mobile Learning: It's here, but what is it?”, *Interactions* 9 (1). Available at: http://www2.warwick.ac.uk/services/ldc/resource/interactions/archive/issue25/ traxler (date of access: 15 November 2015).

Trifanova A. – Ronchetti M. (2003): “Where is mobile learning going?” Proceedings of the E-learn Conference, 1795–1801.

Trifanova A. – Knapp J. – Ronchetti M. – Gamper J. (2004): “Mobile ELDIT: Challenges in the transitions from an e-learning to an m-learning system”. Trento: University of Trento. Available at: http://eprints.biblio.unitn.it/archive/00000532/01/paper4911.pdf (date of access: 17 November 2015).

Turula A. (2015): "Digital TEFL training programmes – in search of a bridge well-balanced", in Turula A. – Chojnacka M. (eds.), 91–110.

Turula, A. – Chojnacka M. (eds.) (2015): *CALL for Bridges between School and Academia, Studies in Computer Assisted Language Learning. Vol. 1*. Frankfurt: Peter Lang.

Ur P. (2009): *A course in language teaching. Practice and theory*. Cambridge: CUP.

Ushioda E. (2001): "Language learning at university: Exploring the role of motivational thinking", in Z. Dörnyei – R. Schmidt (eds.), 91–124.

Vavoula G. – Pachler N. – Kukulska-Hulme A. (eds.) (2009): *Researching mobile learning: Frameworks, tools and research designs*. Oxford: Peter Lang Verlag.

Volet S. – Jarvela S. (eds.) (2001): *Motivation in learning context: Theoretical advances and methodological implications*. Oxford: Elsevier Science Ltd.

Walker K. (2006): "Introduction: Mapping the landscape of mobile learning", in M. Sharples, 3–4.

Wang J. – Liang S. – Ge G. (2008): "Establishment of a medical academic word list", *English for Specific Purposes* 27, 442–58.

Weiner B. (1974): *Achievement motivation and attribution theory*. Morristown, N.J.: General Learning Press.

Wenden A. (1991): *Learner strategies for learner autonomy: Planning and implementing learner training for language learners*. UK: Prentice Hall International.

West R. (1994): "Needs analysis in language teaching", *Language Teaching Abstracts*, 1–19.

Wilkerson M. – Griswold W. – Simon B. (2005): "Ubiquitous presenter: increasing student access and control in a digital lecturing environment", *The 36th SIGCSE technical symposium on computer science education* Vol. 36, 116–120.

Williams M. – Burden R. (1997): *Psychology for language teachers*. Cambridge: Cambridge University Press.

Wilson J. (1986): "General Principles" in D. Harper (ed.), 7–26.

Winters N. (2006): "What is mobile learning", in M. Sharples, 5–9.

Wlodkowski R. (1986): *Enhancing adult motivation to learn*. San Francisco: Jossey-Bass.

Wolters C. (2004): "Advancing achievement goal theory: Using goal structure and goal orientation to predict students' motivation, cognition, and achievement", *Journal of Educational Psychology* 96, 236–250.

Wong L. – Chin C. – Tan C. – Liu M. (2010): "Students' personal and social meaning making in a Chinese idiom mobile learning environment", *Educational Technology and Society* 13(4), 15–26.

Wong L. – Milrad M. – Specht M. (eds.) (2015): Seamless learning in the age of mobile connectivity. Book. Springer-Verlag.

Wood W. (2004): "Clickers: A teaching gimmick that works", *Developmental Cell* 7, 796–798.

Zybert J. (2006): "On (de-)motivating language learners", in J. Zybert (ed.), 194–210.

Zybert J. (2011): "Building learner autonomy through strategy training", SCRIPTA NEOPHILOLOGICA POSNANIENSIA Vol. XI, 133–145.

Zybert J. (2012): *Efektywność w szkolnej nauce języka obcego*. Warszawa: DiG.

Zybert J. (ed.). (2006): Issues in foreign language learning and teaching. Warsaw: Wydawnictwa Uniwersytetu Warszawskiego.

# Appendix A

**<u>Questionnaire 1</u>**

Gender: Male/Female

Why did you choose to study medicine?

- It's a family tradition.
- I want to help others.
- Medicine is my passion.
- Doctors are guaranteed employment after graduation.
- A doctor is a prestigious profession.
- Doctors make good money.

Apart from English, what foreign languages do you know?

Does speaking foreign languages help you learn English for Medical Purposes? If yes, how? If so, how?

In your opinion, success in learning a foreign language depends primarily on:

- Teacher competence
- My motivation to learn
- Appropriate teaching aids
- other _______

What motivates you to learn English for Medical Purposes?

- I want to get a good grade from the language course.
- I want to get to know English better.
- I will benefit from better opportunities on the job market abroad.
- I will benefit from better opportunities on the job market in Poland.
- Specialist literature is mainly in English.
- This will help me in my future career.
- other _______

Which of the following devices do you have?

- a mobile phone/smartphone
- a laptop/netbook computer
- a desktop computer
- a tablet

- an ebook reader
- none of the above

How often do you use social networks (Facebook, Twitter, Instagram, etc.)?

- I'm constantly logged in
- many times a day
- once daily
- 2–3 times a week
- every few weeks
- never

How often do you access the internet/web content on your mobile phone?

- I'm constantly logged in
- many times a day
- once daily
- 2–3 times a week
- every few weeks
- never

How do you access the internet/web content on your mobile phone?

- I have limited data transfer so I'm trying to the use of free wifi whenever possible.
- I have unlimited data transfer.
- I only use free wifi.
- I don't access the internet/web content due to the costs.

Which devices do you use to learn English? And how often (every day, often, i.e. a couple times a week, rarely, i.e. a couple times a month, never).

- a mobile phone/smartphone
- a laptop/netbook computer
- a desktop computer
- a tablet
- an ebook reader
- none of the above

Do you use any particular websites/educational platforms to learn English? If yes, which ones? If not, why not?

Have you ever used any particular computer software to learn English? If yes, which one? If not, why not?

Have you ever used any mobile apps to learn English? If yes, which ones? If not, why not?

Would you be interested in learning English for Medical Purposes via a mobile app?

Apart from regular classes, how much time do you spend learning English for Medical Purposes?

- less than one hour a week
- 1–2 hours a week
- 2–3 hours a week
- over 3 hours a week

Apart from regular classes, when exactly do you usually learn English for Medical Purposes?

Which three features of a mobile learning app do you think are most important?

- low price or being free of charge
- offline use
- personalization of the learning process
- intuitiveness/simplicity of use
- continuity of the learning process
- cross platform use
- ability to adjust to user needs
- possibility to add content
- other _______

Grade the following statements on a scale from 1 to 5 (1 – I strongly disagree, 2 – I disagree to a large extent, 3 – I don't have an opinion, 4 – I agree to a large extent, 5 – I strongly agree).

- Mobile learning makes learning personalized.
- Mobile learning is convenient and effective way of learning.
- In the future, mobile learning will play an important role in English language learning.
- Mobile learning is not an effective way of learning.
- Mobile devices can be a good supplementation of a language course.
- Mobile devices are easy to use.
- A mobile phone is a convenient tool to learn English for Medical Purposes.
- I'm willing to pay for access to a mobile learning platform.
- I prefer mobile devices to a desktop computer.

**Questionnaire 2**

Gender: Male/Female

Did you use Memrise to learn vocabulary from Unit 5? If not, why?

How much time did you spend on learning using Memrise?

- up to 15 minutes
- 15–30 minutes 30 minutes to 1 hour
- 1 hour to 2 hours
- more than 2 hours

When did you use Memrise most often?

Rank Memrise on a scale from 1 to 5 (1 – the lowest grade; 5 – the highest grade). Briefly justify your choice.

Which 3 features of Memrise do you consider most important?

- low price or being free of charge
- offline use
- personalization of the learning process
- intuitiveness/simplicity of use
- continuity of the learning process
- cross platform use
- ability to adjust to user needs
- possibility to add content
- audio files with pronunciation
- other _______

Grade the following statements on a scale from 1 to 5 (1 – I strongly disagree, 2 – I disagree to a large extent, 3 – I don't have an opinion, 4 – I agree to a large extent, 5 – I strongly agree).

- Memrise helped me organize my learning better.
- Memrise made the learning experience more personal.
- Memrise was more convenient to use on a smartphone than on a desktop computer or a laptop/netbook.
- Memrise was more convenient to use on a smartphone than on a tablet.
- I found it convenient that I could use Memrise anywhere at any time.
- A smartphone is a convenient tool for learning English for Medical Purposes.
- I would be willing to upgrade Memrise to a paid version.

- I would recommend Memrise as an educational tool to other medical students.
- I found this way of learning motivating.
- I will use Memrise in the future.
- Compared with traditional paper-based homework, the Memrise exercises were more interesting.
- Thanks to Memrise I learnt more than I would in a traditional way.

What did you like about Memrise?

What didn't you like about Memrise?

What elements would need to changed or introduced to make Memrise better suited to learning English for Medical Purposes?

**Polish Studies in English Language and Literature**

Edited by Jacek Fisiak

Vol. 1 Barbara Lewandowska-Tomaszczyk (ed.): Cognitive Perspectives on Language. 1999.

Vol. 2 Marek Wilczyński: The Phantom and the Abyss. The Gothic Fiction in America and Aesthetics of the Sublime 1798–1856. 1999.

Vol. 3 Ian Firla (ed.): Robert Graves's Historical Novels. 2000.

Vol. 4 Joanna Przedlacka: Estuary English? A Sociophonetic Study of Teenage Speech in the Home Counties. 2002.

Vol. 5 Wiesław Oleksy (ed.): Language Function, Structure, and Change. Essays in Linguistics in Honor of Tomasz P. Krzeszowski. 2002.

Vol. 6 Janusz Arabski (ed.): Time for Words. Studies in Foreign Language Vocabulary Acquisition. 2002.

Vol. 7 Katarzyna Dziubalska-Kołaczyk: Beats-and-Binding Phonology. 2002.

Vol. 8 Zdzisław Wąsik: Epistemological Perspectives on Linguistic Semiotics. 2003.

Vol. 9 Jacek Witkoś: Movement and Reconstruction: Questions and Principle C Effects in English and Polish. 2003.

Vol. 10 Liliana Sikorska (ed.): Aspects of Suffering. Classical Themes in Literature in English. 2004.

Vol. 11 Anna Duszak / Urszula Okulska (eds.): Speaking from the Margin. Global English from a European Perspective. 2004.

Vol. 12 Grzegorz Kość: Robert Lowell. Uncomfortable Epigone of the Grands Maîtres. 2005.

Vol. 13 Liliana Sikorska (ed.): Ironies of Art/Tragedies of Life. Essays on Irish Literature. 2005.

Vol. 14 Urszula Okulska: Gender and the Formation of Modern Standard English. A Socio-Historical Corpus Study with Early Modern English in Focus. 2006.

Vol. 15 Liliana Sikorska (ed.): A Universe of (Hi)Stories. Essays on J.M. Coetzee. 2006.

Vol. 16 Kacper Bartczak: In Search of Communication and Community. The Poetry of John Ashbery. 2006.

Vol. 17 Anna Duszak / Urszula Okulska (eds.): Bridges and Barriers in Metalinguistic Discourse. 2006.

Vol. 18 Arleta Adamska-Sałaciak: Meaning and the Bilingual Dictionary. The Case of English and Polish. 2006.

Vol. 19 Małgorzata Fabiszak (ed.): Language and Meaning. Cognitive and Functional Perspectives. 2007.

Vol. 20 Sabine Heinz: Celtic Literatures – Discoveries. 2007.

Vol. 21 Iwona Kokorniak: English *at*: An Integrated Semantic Analysis. 2007.

Vol. 22 Christina Laurer: Poor Paul: L Vocalisation and the Process of Syllable-Coda Weakening. 2008.

Vol. 23 Jacek Witkoś / Gisbert Fanselow (eds.): Elements of Slavic and Germanic Grammars: A Comparative View. Papers on Topical Issues in Syntax and Morphosyntax. 2008.

Vol. 24 Przemysław Tajsner: Aspects of the Grammar of Focus. A Minimalist View. 2008.

Vol. 25 Ewa Wełnic / Jacek Fisiak (eds.): Friendly Metaphors. Essays on Linguistics, Literature and Culture in Honour of Aleksander Szwedek. 2008.

Vol. 26 Michał Janowski: Inheritance of Features in Metaphoric Mappings in English. 2009.

Vol. 27 Cognitive Approaches to Language and Linguistic Data. Studies in honor of Barbara Lewandowska-Tomaszczyk. Edited by Wiesław Oleksy and Piotr Stalmaszczyk. 2009.

Vol. 28 Andrzej Kopcewicz: Intertextual Transactions in American and Irish Fictions. Edited by Janusz Semrau. 2009.

Vol. 29 Janusz Semrau (ed.): "Will you tell me *any thing* about yourself?" Comemorative Essays on Herman Meville's "Bartleby the Scrivener". 2009.

Vol. 30 Minako Nakayasu: The Pragmatics of Modals in Shakespeare. 2009.

Vol. 31 Magdalena Wrembel / Małgorzata Kul / Katarzyna Dziubalska-Kołaczyk (eds.): Achievements and Perspectives in SLA of Speech: New Sounds 2010. Volume I. 2011.

Vol. 32 Magdalena Wrembel / Małgorzata Kul / Katarzyna Dziubalska-Kołaczyk (eds.): Achievements and Perspectives in SLA of Speech: New Sounds 2010. Volume II. 2011.

Vol. 33 Anna Turula: Form-Focused Instruction and the Advanced Language Learner. On the Importance of the Semantics of Grammar. 2011.

Vol. 34 Sylwia Wojciechowska: Conceptual Metonymy and Lexicographic Representation. 2012.

Vol. 35 Hanna Rutkowska: Orthographic Systems in Thirteen Editions of the *Kalender of Shepherdes* (1506–1656). 2013.

Vol. 36 Natalia Budohoska: English in Kenya or Kenyan English? 2014.

Vol. 37 Maria Dakowska: In Search of Processes of Language Use in Foreign Language Didactics. 2015.

Vol. 38 Beata Wyszyńska: Language Therapy Space. Teaching English as a Foreign Language to the Visually Impaired. 2016.

Vol. 39 Maria Chojnacka: Optimizing the Process of Teaching English for Medical Purposes with the Use of Mobile Applications. A Memrise-based Case Study. 2017.

www.peterlang.com

www.ingramcontent.com/pod-product-compliance
Ingram Content Group UK Ltd.
Pitfield, Milton Keynes, MK11 3LW, UK
UKHW011005120926
8556IPUK00027B/74

9 783631 730614